BACK TO THE
House of Health 2

BACK TO THE
House of Health 2

MORE REJUVENATING RECIPES TO
Alkalize and Energize for Life!

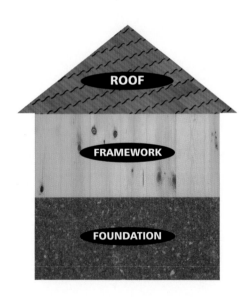

Shelley Redford Young, L.M.T.

Foreword and Diabetic Research by Robert O. Young, Ph.D., D.Sc.

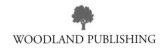

WOODLAND PUBLISHING

BACK TO THE
House of Health 2

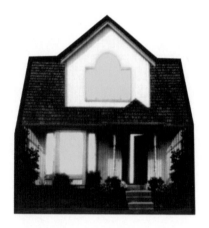

ISBN 1-58054-377-4

Published by Woodland Publishing
448 East 800 North
Orem, Utah 84097
(800) 777-2665
www.woodlandpublishing.com

Photography by Stefan Hallberg

Printed in the United States of America.

Note: The information in this book is for educational purposes only and is not recommended as a means of diagnosing or treating an illness. All matters concerning physical and mental health should be supervised by a health practitioner knowledgeable in treating that particular condition. Neither the publisher nor author directly or indirectly dispense medical advice, nor do they prescribe any remedies or assume any responsibility for those who choose to treat themselves.

Contents

Recipe Titles by Alphabetical Order

Recipe Titles by Category

Acknowledgments

I remember, about 15 years ago, when Robert and I started the InnerLight Company. I never dreamed that I would be guided to help people with the diet/lifestyle portion of this mission. I had always avoided the kitchen. After all, if I was stuck in the kitchen, I would miss everything out there in the exciting world, right?

Now I love the kitchen because it is a healing, artistic place. I love getting the new research from Robert (Dr. Young) and others, and then creating healing masterpieces that will allow people more time out in their exciting world. It's very cool to paint with God's palette.

I want to thank Robert, aka: Dr. Dust, Za Chosen Von ;) wink, the King of Health, or in his own words, the Messenger, for his never ending love, faith and confidence in me. When I met Rob at the tender age of 15, (yes, he robbed the cradle ☺) I really didn't realize what a journey we had ahead of us, and I can tell you, it has been exciting to be out in the world with him.☺

My children continue to be the LIGHTS of my life, and now with our daughter Ashley Rose (24) teaching her own Yoga and Alkalarian cooking classes, and our son-in-law, Matthew (27), who creates InnerLight-Motion, our message can come into your home every week. What a blessing! Young parents teaching their child (CharLee Bear) and others to Alkalize and Energize! We CAN help the next generation! And it's worth it!

I believe Walt Disney's statement: *"Our greatest natural resource is the minds of our children."*

My sons Adam (27) (in Chicago) and Andrew (19) (in Brazil) are also helping others with their example and knowledge and I want to thank them for being such great sons, true friends, and supporters. To Alex (15 and still transitioning ☺) who remains here on the Ranch AvoRado, with Mammus and Paps... I want you to know that I know all this has been such a hard act to follow and you have been and continue to be, a great joy for Rob and I. Thank you for being our gentle caboose and for eating at least half of everything I make ;) wink ☺

Elizabeth Stowe said: *"Making the decision to have a child—It's momentous. It is to decide forever to have your heart go walking around outside your body."*

And so to all of my children: My heart is with you! xoxo

Back to the House of Health 2 has been created from truly a Gift of Givers, in that it is a wonderful collection of recipes from many Alkalarian chefs who entered our annual pH Miracle Recipe Contest (July 2003) and agreed to have their recipes published along with mine to make this recipe book a synergistic showing of Alkalarian ART! The support and offerings from the contest was so incredibly creative and generous! People who cared enough to share and give of their masterpieces so that all could enjoy and benefit. Thank you from the bottom of my heart for taking the time to send in your healing recipes. You will now have many many people all around the world applauding you as I do! ☺ Some of the winners, won pH Miracle Retreats and it has been so wonderful for Rob and I to honor you and get to know you! Thank you FRIENDS.

Special thanks goes out to a new angel of Light in my life, Donna Downing (a feeder of sheep too☺). To Donna and also to our dear friend, Dr. Gloria Ma, thanks for helping me prepare the recipes from the contest and helping us judge the contest. I trust you and your tastebuds.☺

To our great InnerLight Foundation support team, Ryan and Ashley Thayne. Thank you! We love you two! Thank you for all you do to help us at the Ranch AvoRado and for giving life and breath to Doc Broc and the AvoRado Kid at our pH Miracle Retreats. Ashley, thanks for the help in proofing the book and for all the follow-up with the winners of the pH Miracle recipe contest.

A full color recipe book doesn't just happen. It takes a great crew of people who support and aid you in your efforts. It also takes the faith of a good publisher. My gratitude to Woodland Publishing for once again, getting this recipe book out in record time! For my talented photographer, who made himself available, to render this beautiful food, once again, in perfect Light. Thank you Stephan Hallberg!

To a sister ☺ Jillair Meine, for her tireless hours of staging, and set designing the shots so they sing! And thank you for the use of your beautiful dishes and props that made the pictures so pretty, just like you! Thank you, Thank you, Thank you xoxoxo

Sincere thanks goes to my other family members, and friends who helped during the shooting of this book, with prepping and preparing the food trays: Lori Lisonbee, (CharLee Bear's other alkalarian Grandma) Brock, Amber, and Aspen (baby on cover) Doxey and sweet Matthew and Ashley Rose and CharLee Bear. I couldn't have done it without your love and support! And thank you also to all my great models who really showed how great you can look when you eat Alkalarian! Thanks Lee and Whitney Lisonbee! I'm so glad we're family!☺

To my Heavenly Father and my Savior, Jesus Christ: Thank you for guiding me, and showing me Your ways, wisdom, and intent for Your sheep. Thank you for allowing me to paint with your incredible palette in my kitchen. Thank you for my own health and strength and the chance to serve those who have lost their way from Your House of Health. Thank you for raising up friends, satellites, (distributors) who help us get this good news and hope out into the world! For all YOUR healing creations and all YOUR unconditional love, I am grateful.

In continued light and love,

Shelley

Foreword

Your body seeks to maintain a balance in a number of different factors. Your temperature is an example of one such balance. Your body tries to maintain a temperature of 98.6° Fahrenheit. Variances of only a few degrees above or below can result in serious problems and even death, but there is one balance that is more crucial than any other—the balance between acids and bases.

Your body will go to great measures to maintain its slightly basic or alkaline level, especially in the blood. Overacidification of the body sets you up for sickness. In the slightly alkaline environment of a healthy body, germs cannot thrive and therefore cannot cause problems. However, an acidic environment is exactly what these germs are looking for. In such an environment they can thrive and cause illness.

Additionally, as the body changes from alkaline to acidic, other organisms start causing problems. Your body naturally has some microorganisms present in it—many are necessary for life functions. Normally your body can keep these microorganisms in check, but when you lose your balance these microorganisms can gain the upper hand and start causing problems.

The relationship between acids and alkalines is quantified by a pH measurement. Based on a scale of one to fourteen, with seven being neutral, pH measures the acidic or alkaline level. When acids and alkalines meet in certain ratios, they neutralize each other. Your body actually seeks to maintain a pH level of 7.365, which is slightly alkaline. With the exception of certain body systems—specifically the stomach and colon—your body will try to maintain that pH level.

Physiological disease is actually a manifestation of an imbalance in the pH level of your body fluids. As your body becomes more and more acidic, it will send out red flags to let you know that you need to return to a balanced state. The imbalance between acids and alkalines is in your control.

Your body had a defense mechanism already in place to help maintain it pH balance. Certain substances found in our foods are alkaline in nature—such as sodium, potassium, calcium. and magnesium. Your body keeps minerals like these in stores for when your pH level starts to turn acidic. When problems start, these stores are opened up and the body's pH level is returned to normal.

But if there are insufficient levels of these minerals, then your body will start pulling them from other areas like the bones—for calcium; or from muscles—for the magnesium. The problem is that these areas need those minerals too, and are weakened by the gleaning that your body is forced to do in order to maintain pH balance.

There's nothing complicated about eating to maintain good health, energy, vitality and fitness. Eat plenty of less acidic food, and skip the acidic foods. You need to eat lots of green vegetables, good alkaline water, like from young coconuts, and good fats. You need to not eat sugars and starches. You need to eat frequently, and you need to stop eating when you are satisfied.

That's it!

Follow the guidelines and eat and drink the alkaline recipes in this book, and all your cells will be able to get and use all the energy they need without getting overwhelmed by the acids produced from sugar and protein.

Disease like diabetes (the fastest growing illness in the world today) and a host of other health problems will become a thing of the past. Just remember when you fill up your tank with Shelley's recipes, you will be using premium. Don't bother with the junk; stick with nature's wholesome bounty for glowing good health.

A decade-long study of Type I diabetes found that those who kept their blood sugar levels near normal cut their risk of eye, kidney and nerve damage up to 70 percent. Uncontrolled sugar levels, however, increased the risk of blindness, heart disease, stroke, kidney failure, nerve damage, skin problems and more. The landmark 2001 NIH clinical trail Diabetes Prevention Program showed conclusively that diet and exercise slash the risk of Type 2 diabetes by up to 58 percent. And that's with a very conventional diet approach.

Shelley has made it even easier to eat more alkaline and less acidic with her latest and greatest recipes. In fact, my own 15 years of experience and research and two recent controlled studies show that Shelley's recipe plan does even better: it cuts the risk 100 percent. And it prevents and reverses not only Type II diabetes, but Type I as well.

Furthermore, the type and quality of the fuel you put into your body determines whether or not you "graduate" from hypo/hyperglycemia to diabetes. An acidic diet will eventually push the body right over the borderline, while an alkaline diet will save you from ever hearing that diagnosis.

All that thanks mainly to Shelley's alkaline recipes that incorporate greens and good fats.

The underlying idea of Shelley's new recipes is to teach your body to burn fat for energy rather than sugar or protein. Fat is a much cleaner fuel, and doesn't leave behind the toxic acidic wastes sugar and protein metabolism does. Using recipes with good fat offers the body the opportunity to burn fat which gives the pancreas a break, and allows the body to begin healing the pancreas and its insulin-producing beta cells. That is why Shelley's revolutionary recipes can prevent and reverse diabetes as well as heart disease and the

other negative effects brought on from a diet high in sugar and protein.

As you start eating and drinking a more alkaline diet from over one-hundred new recipes contained in this book, you will begin to experience physical change. You should also know that as you change for the better physically, you will be improving psychologically as well; one feeds right into the other, on a two-way street, As you grow both physically and emotionally stronger, you will begin thinking better, and you will do better—and you will be able to connect to your true self. And that, my friends, is spiritually, though it may come in a thousand disguises.

This is the key to ultimate health, fitness, energy, vitality, love, joy, and happiness. All a gift from our Creator delivered through an incredibly beautiful, talented, artistic and spiritual woman, I have had the honor and privilege of living and working with, as my eternal companion, for over thirty years.

I know you will enjoy the taste and flavor as well as the healthy benefits of each new recipe, as I have in the past and continue to enjoy on a daily basis.

It is my honor now to give you Shelley Redford Young and co-contributors of which we are eternally grateful, "Back to the House of Health 2" and over one-hundred incredibly new and delicious alkalizing recipes that will change your life forever.

In Love and InnerLight,

Dr. Robert O. Young
Husband, Father and Research Scientist

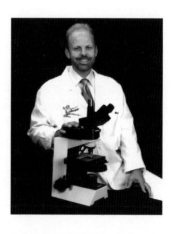

Preface

Ahem...:)   My Fellow Alkalarians, :D (soy-cheeser grin)

I approach you all, once again, being overwhelmed with the deepest gratitude for the healing gifts from our truly concerned and caring Creator. As I continue to witness pH Miracles all around the world, I know that out in our Universe, there is, (as Mr. Rogers stated), a heart that beats, which loves and cares for each and every one of us. Our Heavenly Father, who wants the best for all of us. I know this to be TRUE, because the garden was here before we were. Someone planted and placed it, and put it all around us to whisper, I am here and always have been.... for you.

With more research coming in everyday about God's Garden being the very best medicine cabinet we can have in our homes, I am reminded time after time, that the way to build good cells is to build good blood. As Dr. Dust (Robert O. Young) states: "The way to build good blood, is through the best blood transfusion in the world, the Greens."

I've always known, that Avocado was God's butter, but to have new research sent to us, with studies from Oxford University in Britain, proving that an extract from Avocados called mannoheptulose, is showing promise as a new cancer adjunct, inhibiting the growth rate of tumor cell lines, is so exciting and so confirming. The fact that Avocados inhibit glycolysis, a fermentation of glucose, which cancer cells thrive in, is once again a reminder that we all need to stay very close to the protective and healing organic garden.

Also, this year we were blessed to be placed in the middle of an avocado grove, Ranch AvoRado (of course ;) wink...Y'all come on out and see us now... ya heah!☺ To have this beautiful place to share with those who want to learn more and experience more about the New Biology, has truly gone beyond our wildest dreams to reach out and touch others—to lift them with LIGHT. The fact that a beautiful row of grass was planted (before we arrived) between two rows of 7 palms is no coincidence to us. It was a sign that we were in the right place at the right time.

With more positive research and study at the cellular level, we have added some other foods and herbs to our lineup offering in this, the 2nd edition of *Back to the House of Health*. Clinical studies have shown that coconut oil has anti-microbial and anti-viral properties. Rich in lauric oils that are 2nd only to those found in a perfectly balanced food, mother's milk. And remember when Tom Hanks survived so beautifully on coconuts and fresh coconut water in the movie, Castaway? It got me thinking, and I ran some fresh coconut water into Dr. Young and asked him to test the pH of it. Any guesses?..... 7.36... hmmm the same pH as our own blood streams. Now our favorite thirst quenching treat is a glass of Young coconut water. You gotta try it!!!! The coconut meat of young coconuts is also a hidden treasure of alkalizing buffers to neutralize acidity.. they being phosphorus, calcium, iron, caprilic and capric fats.☺ There are several great recipes using these wonderful gifts from the islands. Dr. Young has also included them in his Diabetes controlled study and found amazing success.

Also, in Dr. Young's Diabetes research, he found enough evidence to feel good about allowing Stevia into the Alkalarian program in moderation. Yippie! Finally a safe sweetener. This has opened the door to creating new breakfast shakes and some Alkalarian desserts that are wonderfully packed with healthy fats (avocados, coconut waters, and fresh silky almond milk) and a subtle sweetness that makes them yummie but not playing havoc with our health. We even have a pudding and popcicles (see front cover) made with Soy Sprouts and Stevia.... now that's progress!☺ To read even more great research on Stevia and Coconut Oil, check out *The pH Miracles of Diabetes*, AOL Time Warner Publisher.

We held the first annual pH Miracle Recipe contest (July 2003) and you are now the lucky recipient of many wonderful, soothing, delicious dishes from many gracious alkalarian chefs. The creativity has been over the top! Vegan Chili with the chili sauce made from salad greens ... Avocado Key Lime Pie and even a China Moon Thai dish that has many sauce variations!!! I'm sure you'll appreciate the different ways these new dishes are seasoned and presented. We are all so blessed, aren't we?☺ Thank you my fellow Alkalarian chefs! xoxo

And finally, I am so pleased to witness the evolution of the old acidic food pyramid into a real alkalizing healing symbol. Dr. Young decided it should literally be a House of Health, not a pyramid anymore. The House of Health is more fitting and will teach our children about their own temples (their bodies) and how to keep that house healthy and strong and how to keep their own rivers and streams running clean and pure. We've all been invited to make this change and it's happening . . . I'm assured that this change is here to stay.☺

In gratitude and continued faith in HIM who feeds us all!

Shelley Redford Young

Further InLightenment

(Please refer to the first edition of the Back to the House of Health recipe book for introductory information on "The New Biology," acid/alkaline diet guidelines, food combining, transitional and phasing ideas, Shelley's shortcuts, glossary terms, and valuable pH nutritional charts and tables.)

Let Your Medicine be Your Food

"Let your food be your medicine and your medicine be your food."
Hippocrates

I love the simplicity of Hippocrates' counsel, and I love realizing that the food that has been provided for us from the Garden is simply that which will keep us all well.

The Alkalarian diet and lifestyle does an important balancing act in our bloodstream, which is the river of life. This balancing act is needed by everyone, not just someone suffering from the extreme imbalance of diabetes, heart disease, or cancer (which are in epidemic proportions now). It is important for all of us to learn how to prevent those states of imbalance. We need to discover the causes of disease and learn how to prevent them in our own bodies.

Dr. Robert O. Young has said: "It is in the *prevention of disease* that we will truly find the cure."

I am anxious for the next generation (our children and their children) to learn about the pH scale and its importance to the cells, fluids and tissues of our bodies. Once they understand this, I think it will make the decision of choosing foods that are beneficial for us easier. They will eat for health, not just for pleasure, and we all know that food can taste good but not be good for us. I

believe God's healing foods can also taste great once we achieve a balanced blood terrain, and once our taste buds have been adjusted to the subtle, humble sweetness of vegetables. Once our kids start eating and drinking alkaline (following our example), they will be building and contributing to their health physically and psychologically.

By normalizing blood sugar and slowing down or eliminating the process of glycolysis (a fermentation of glucose/sugar which acidic cancer cells thrive in), the risks to our long-term health prospects decrease, and a lot of stress is removed from our systems. We can make energy deposits, not withdrawals, every time we dine alkaline. Eating an alkalarian diet can be the best preventative measure we can take to avoid ever coming down with a serious degenerative disease. The first step in eating an alkalarian diet is to keep a balanced blood sugar level.

Normalizing blood sugar and maintaining a balanced bloodstream involves these eight basic rules:

1) Eliminate all foods that contain moderate or high levels of sugar, including high-sugar fruits like apples, bananas, cherries, etc. which contain sugar (fructose). When such fruits are introduced into a yeast-ridden blood terrain, they can cause havoc. Other foods that should be eliminated from our diets are: grains (maltose) such as wheat, rice, or oats; dairy (lactose), such as milk, cheese, yogurt,

13

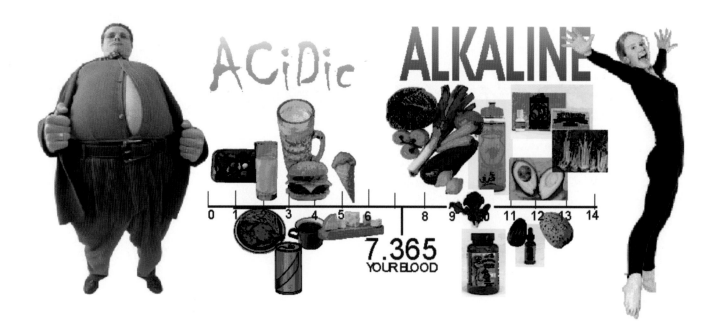

or ice cream (one of the major contributors to diabetes); processed sugar (sucrose); and starchy foods like potatoes and breads.

2) Limit your carbohydrate intake to low carbohydrates such as spinach, parsley, broccoli, celery, cucumber, leafy greens, seaweeds, grasses and low-sugar fruits like avocado, tomatillos, lemon, lime, red and green peppers, and low-sugar grapefruit. These foods can be eaten freely.

3) Eat liberal amounts of good fats from avocados (God's butter), marine oils (from salmon, trout, tuna, cod, etc.), flax oil, borage oil, hemp oil, primrose oil, olive oil, or mixed oils, like Essential Balance Oil from Arrowhead Mills, Omega Nutrition or Udo's oil. Also coconut oil, milk, and water are making a great come back. We are rediscovering the benefits of the naturally occurring fats and minerals in unprocessed coconuts and raw coconut water—which has the same pH as our blood, 7.36.

4) Hydrate with alkaline water that has a pH of 8.0 or above and at least one liter per 30 pounds of weight. This would also include fresh green juices or water with one teaspoon of concentrated green power, with 16 drops of sodium chlorite or sodium silicate. (Refer to Dr. Young's books, *Sick and Tired*, *The pH Miracle* and *The pH Miracle for Diabetes* for more information on this.)

5) Take nutritional supplements that will support and help balance the bloodstream. In other words—reclaim your inner terrain!

6) Stop eating when you no longer feel hunger (once you are satisfied) and not when you are stuffed. Eat smaller, more frequent meals that consist of alkaline-based recipes like those in *Back to House of Health* and in this second edition. Remember the foundational rule for healthy living and eating: less is more and more is less, and less more often is better than more less often. Learn to visually keep your meals to a 70/30 or 80/20 ratio when building your plate. (Refer to *Back to the House of Health* for dietary guidelines, transitional ideas, pantry inventories, Shelley's shortcuts, and food-combining rules.)

7) Exercise! Get out and walk. MOVE your body! Swim, hike, bike, dance, run, lift weights, take yoga or an aerobics class. Stretch and breathe deeply—your lymphatic system will thank you.

Exercise and breathing are essential to help the body eliminate toxic acids that can build up as a result of poor eating, little or no exercise, emotional disturbances, lack of rest or depression.

8) Get good rest. A good night's sleep where the body experiences deep restful REM sleep allows the body to revive, repair and regenerate. If you often wake up in the middle of the night it may mean an emotional issue is surfacing from your subconscious, or it may mean you have adrenal exhaustion or some other physical health issue. Try to keep stress to a minimum and live, eat, and think in a way that will bring you true peace of mind.

These foundational eight steps will help you in controlling, balancing and normalizing blood sugar levels. Another important aspect in controlling sugar levels is Dr. Young's new Food pyramid. Actually it's not a pyramid at all . . . it's a HOUSE OF HEALTH.

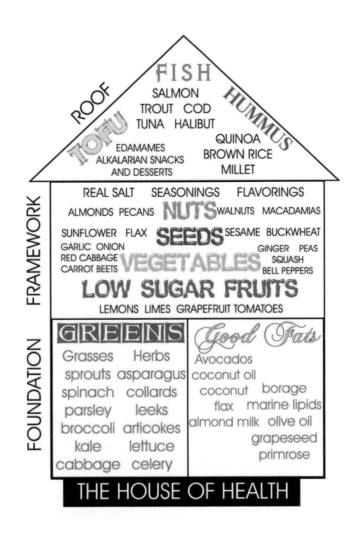

From Dr. Robert O. Young:

A New Food Pyramid–
The House of Health

The new food pyramid is not a pyramid at all, but a house—A House of Health. This is a House that views life from all aspects: physical, emotional and spiritual. If we are to achieve ultimate health, fitness and vitality, we must balance our lives in ALL aspects. It is important to understand that the physical affects the emotional, and the emotional affects the physical. The physical affects the spiritual and the spiritual affects the physical. The emotional affects the spiritual and the spiritual affects the emotional. I call this the triad of life. Our levels of physical, emotional and spiritual health are all interconnected. As we look at the House of Health from this point of view then I would suggest that the foundation of our House is physical, the framework is our emotional state and the roof that caps our House is spiritual. Each part of the House is essential and connected to the other. For us to enjoy optimal physical, emotional and spiritual health the focus must begin with the foundation, the physical. This is because the physiology of our body will affect the psychology and the psychology will affect the physiology.

As we contemplate the USDA Food Pyramid (see right), we must realize that its emphasis is on foods that will not bring us ultimate health and vitality. Such foods include acidic foods such as breads, cereals, rice, pasta, high-sugar fruits, meats, dairy, and sweets. The foundation of health and vitality in the House of Health is created by a very different array of foods. The House of Health is divided into three parts: the foundation, the framework and the roof.

The Foundation

The House of Health is founded on all the good fats, such as avocado, coconut oil, flax, borage, hemp, olive, and primrose oil. This foundation also includes green foods like wheat grass, barley grass, celery, spinach, celery, broccoli, cabbage

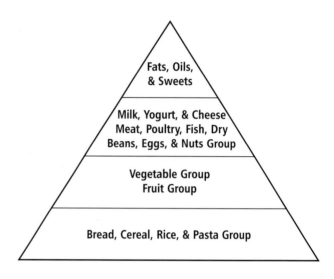

USDA Food Pyramid (acid forming)

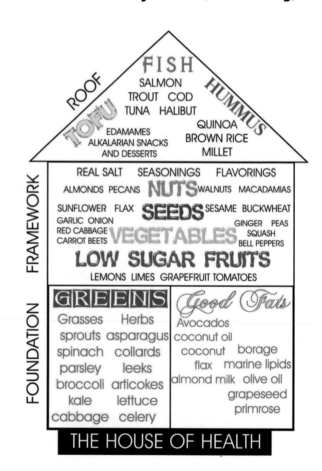

parsley, leafy greens and sprouts. These and other green foods, green drinks, and good fats form the foundation of the House of Health. These foods will provide proper alkaline context for pH balanced body fluids and the foundational anatomical elements–the microzymas-that will build healthy blood cells, which in turn will build our body cells.

The Framework

The framework of the House of Health includes nuts (almonds, pecans, walnuts and hazelnuts), seeds (sesame, buckwheat, and flax), root vegetables (garlic, ginger, jicama and onion) and all the low-sugar fruits (lemon, lime, grapefruit, bell peppers, and tomatoes). These foods will help neutralize acids and keep our body fluids pH balanced.

The Roof

Finally, the roof of the House of Health should include fish (salmon, trout, tuna, halibut, swordfish, mackerel) and soy products (tofu and edamame). These foods also contain the foundational fats and proteins that the body needs as it creates cellular structure.

As you move to the House of Health by eating a more alkaline diet, you will begin to experience a change in your physiology. As your physiology improves, your psychology will improve, and as your psychology improves you will begin to connect to your true self, or your spirituality. As you start feeling better, you will start thinking better, and as you start feeling and thinking better you will start doing better. The key to ultimate health, fitness, energy, vitality, joy, love and happiness can be found when you go home, home to the House of Health. Start today by eating better and begin living the principles of the "pH Miracle Lifestyle and Diet."

Latest Research on God's Healing Gifts

God's Butter: Avocado

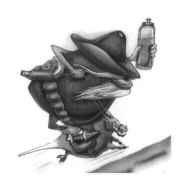

The AvoRado Kid on his Horseradish Lightning

Avocados are rich in nutrients, with vitamins A, B-complex, C, E, H, K and folic acid. They also contain the buffering minerals so critical in neutralizing excess acidity, magnesium, copper, iron, calcium, potassium, and many other trace elements.

Avocados are a perfect food in that they provide all of the essential amino acids—18 aminos in all—plus 7 fatty acids, including Omega 3 and 6. They also contain more protein than cow's milk, (about 2 percent per edible portion. (For more information, see "The Protein/Calcium Myth" in Back to the House of Health.)

The water content of an avocado ranges from 65-80 percent. This high water content makes an avocado a type of hydrating and energizing fuel for the body to burn, instead of a sugar-based fuel which leaves acidic ash waste in our blood. The avocado ranks as the most easily digested rich source of fats and proteins in a whole food. Approximately 63 percent of the fat contained in avocado is monounsaturated, and only 17 percent is saturated. Both types of fat serve as good energy sources in the body once we convert to fat as the source for our fuel (rather than sugars and high proteins). The rest of the fat found in an avocado, about 20 percent, is polyunsaturated and serves in cell construction.

Scientific evidence from a May 1999 study conducted by the California Avocado Commission shows that nutrient-dense avocados contain 76 mg of beta-sitosterol per 100 grams of fruit. Beta-sitosterol is a plant sterol that occurs naturally in the avocado. Certain sterols can inhibit cholesterol absorption in the intestine and result in lower blood cholesterol levels. For example, in animal studies, phytosterol (in the form of beta-sitosterol) has been shown to inhibit the growth of tumors, particularly the growth of prostate tumors. Beta-sitosterol is incredibly beneficial to health. The 76 mg found in avocados is more than four times the level found in other commonly eaten fruits, such as bananas, apples, cantaloupes, grapes, plums and cherries. And avocados do not have all the sugar that raises blood glucose! Avocados also contain at least twice the amount of beta-sitosterol found in other foods, including corn, green soybeans and olives.

A survey conducted by the National Cancer Institute in a 1992 demonstrated that ounce per ounce, the glutathione content of avocados is three times that of bananas, apples, cantaloupes, grapes, plums and cherries. Glutathione is composed of three amino acids and functions as a buffer, neutralizing acids that can cause damage to cells in the body during the process of aging, heart disease and cancer. Numerous studies have linked glutathione to the prevention of various types of cancer, including cancer of the mouth and pharynx, and also heart disease.

Dr. David Heber, director of the UCLA Center for Human Nutrition and author of *What Color Is Your Diet,* has this to say about avocados: "The California avocado is an excellent dietary source of glutathione and phytosterol, further demonstrating the value of the diverse plant-based diet in providing micronutrients that may have unique roles in the body and the potential to improve overall health and prevent chronic disease."

Dr. Heber's findings also indicate that avocados contain a biochemical called lutein, a carotenoid recently discovered in avocados and found in green vegetables, which can help protect against various forms of cancer, including prostate cancer. UCLA lab tests showed that lutein reduces

prostate cancer cell growth by 25 percent, while lycopene from tomatoes reduces cell growth by 20 percent. When lutein and lycopene were combined, prostate cancer cell growth was reduced by 32 percent. This indicates that both nutrients together help protect against prostate cancer better than either nutrient alone. "Lutein and lycopene in combination appear to have additive or synergistic effects against prostate cancer," said Heber. "Our results suggest that further study should be done to investigate the nutrient interactions of lutein and lycopene at a subcellular and molecular level."

Traditionally, lutein has been found in green vegetables such as parsley, celery and spinach, but it was also recently discovered in avocados. In fact, research shows that avocados are the highest fruit source of lutein among the 20 most frequently consumed fruits. In addition to the new prostate cancer findings, lutein is also known to protect against eye diseases such as cataracts and macular degeneration, the leading cause of blindness in the elderly.

The new research at UCLA also indicates that avocados have nearly twice as much vitamin E as previously reported, making avocados the highest fruit source of this powerful buffer of acid. Vitamin E is known to slow the aging process and to protect against heart disease and common forms of cancer by neutralizing acids, which may cause cellular damage. Dr. David Heber states, "Avocados are recognized as an excellent source of monounsaturated fat which is known to lower cholesterol levels, but the antioxidant and biochemical properties of avocados are less well-recognized. These plant nutrients naturally found in fruits and vegetables work together to reduce oxidative stress and prevent disease."

Dr. Heber, along with 35 scientists at the UCLA Center for Human Nutrition, has long endorsed a diet based on 5 to 11 servings per day of a diverse selection of fruits and vegetables, including the avocado. Worldwide research demonstrates the high intake of fruits and vegetables is associated with better health, largely due to their disease-fighting properties.

The avocado also contains fourteen minerals,

all of which regulate body functions and stimulate growth. Especially noteworthy are its levels of iron and copper. These minerals aid in red blood cell regeneration and the prevention of nutritional anemia. Avocados are also a higher source of potassium than bananas, and contain sodium, which gives them a high alkaline reaction without all the sugar. Avocados contain no starch and very little sugar and therefore do not raise blood sugar levels but provide a high source of fat, which the body can metabolize for energy and use for construction of cellular membranes. The avocado is also a great source of protein at 10 to 15 percent.

For all the reasons above, the avocado will be one of the most important foods that you eat as you balance your blood sugar levels. Dr. Young encourages anyone suffering from Type 1 or Type 2 diabetes to eat avocados liberally so that the body moves away from sugar metabolism to fat metabolism. This will allow the body to enjoy the protective attributes of the "pH Miracle Lifestyle and Diet." One of our favorite avocado breakfasts is the AvoRado Kid Super Greens Shake found on page 35 or the Zippy Breakfast found in *Back to the House of Health*. Or try the new Avocado Key Lime Pie on page 109. For beautiful organically grown California avocados picked fresh off the tree and shipped to you, contact: www.ranchavorado.com

Lemons, Limes and Grapefruits

Many people think that lemons, limes and grapefruits are acidic fruits, but they are not. They have an alkaline ash after digestion. Their potassium and sodium content is metabolized to bicarbonate and therefore alkalizes not acidifies the blood and tissues. You can use lemon or lime in all the fluids you drink to help alkalize your body fluids and maintain their delicate pH balance.

The Awesome Tomato

The tomato is not acidic because of its low sugar content and is alkaline forming when it enters the bloodstream. It increases the alkalinity of the blood and helps remove acids, especially uric and sulphuric acid (which come from eating meat). In this way tomatoes help to balance blood pH levels. As a liver cleanser, tomatoes are wonderful and can be used in raw vegetable juices or soups. My favorite is the Madrid Gazpacho soup from *The pH Miracle*, or the Rich Raw Tomato Sauce in *Back to the House of Health*. Also try the Creamy Tomato Soup on page 51 in this book. Just another word of advice, eat lots of fresh, whole tomatoes. This does not include processed tomatoes like canned or bottled tomato sauces or even canned tomato juice, because they are acidic.

Another incredible benefit from eating tomatoes is their high concentration of a newfound nutrient called lycopene. Lycopenes are part of the family of pigments called carotenoids, which are natural compounds that create the colors of fruits and vegetables. For example, beta carotene is the orange pigment in carrots. Lycopene is the substance that makes tomatoes red. Similar to essential amino acids, lycopenes are not made in the human body. My research indicates that lycopenes, for the most part, are buffers of acids in the human body.

In December 1995, the *Journal of the National Cancer Institute* published the results of a study conducted by Harvard University researchers. This study showed an association between consuming a diet rich in tomatoes and a decreased risk of prostate cancer. The researchers surveyed the eating habits of over 47,000 men between the ages of 40 and 75 for six years and found that the men who consumed more tomatoes were at a lower risk for prostate cancer. Researchers theorize that lycopene may be responsible for this possible protective effect.

In another study on tomatoes done in March of 1999, results suggest that the consumption of lycopene may prevent cancer. Omer Kucak, M.D., oncologist at the Barbara Ann Karmanos Cancer Institute in Detroit, conducted the research which indicates that lycopene supplements containing tomato extract may protect against prostate cancer.

In the study, Dr. Kucak and colleagues followed 30 men with localized prostate cancer who were scheduled to undergo surgical removal of the prostate. For three weeks prior to surgery, study participants were randomly assigned to receive either a 15 mg capsule of lycopene as a pure tomato extract, twice daily, or no intervention. On removal of the prostate, the glands were analyzed to determine whether there were any differences between the two groups studied.

Investigators found that the group treated with lycopene supplements had smaller tumors and the cancer was more frequently confined to the prostate, meaning the cancer did not spread to surrounding tissue and organs. Levels of serum PSA (prostate specific antigen, a common marker used to detect prostate cancer) actually declined during the three-week span that participants took the lycopene supplements. In addition, the tumors in participants who consumed lycopene showed signs of regression and decreased malignancy.

"This study represents the first clinical evidence that lycopene in supplements may prevent cancer," said Dr. Kucak. "Furthermore, the findings suggest that lycopene may not only help prevent cancer, but may also be useful in treating men who are already diagnosed with prostate cancer."

For more information about the study call Karmanos Cancer Institute at (313) 745-4226 or visit the Institute's website: www.Karmanos.org.

Cuckoo about Coconuts

For over 3,000 years the coconut has been cultivated in Southern Asia and the East Indian islands. The coconut palm is found all along tropical coasts and its fruit is used as the principal food on many of the Pacific islands. You may have seen Tom Hanks, seriously overweight, in the movie Castaway. He was stranded on an island drinking coconut water, eating coconut milk and fresh fish and losing weight and getting strong and healthy. Sounds like a good idea!

A few years, ago, a successful campaign was carried out through the media to scare Americans away from coconut milk and coconut oils. The claim was made that the fat content of coconut contributed to heart disease, so businesses and consumers were urged replace coconut oils with hydrogenated vegetable oils. Dr. C. Everett Koop,

former Surgeon General of the United States, called the scare of tropical foods like coconuts "foolishness."

The problem with any food is in its processing. A food high in saturated and monounsaturated fats, such as coconut, is greatly affected by refining. When coconut is refined and hydrogenated, the oil chains cross-link and create what science calls trans-fats. These trans-fats, not the naturally occurring fats, lead to circulation challenges and have been implicated in causing arteriosclerosis. The whole, unprocessed oils found in coconut prior to the refining do not pose such a danger. In fact, there are studies that show that the fat found in coconut actually helps lower cholesterol and thus prevents arteriosclerosis and heart disease.

In 1982, research scientists Kaunitz and Dayrit showed that islanders with a high intake of coconut oil showed no evidence of the harmful effects often associated with the high intake of saturated fat. When some of the islanders migrated to New Zealand however, and lowered their intake of coconut oil, their total cholesterol and LDL cholesterol increased, and their HDL cholesterol decreased.

Coconut milk is made from the fruit itself, by liquefying the white meat. Coconut milk can be compared to a mother's breast milk in its chemical balance. It is also a complete protein food at 15 percent, when taken in its natural form. The milk is an excellent source of phosphorus, calcium, and iron. Most importantly, coconuts are 70 percent fat. Of that fat, 90 percent is medium-chain triglyceride saturated fat and 10 percent is monounsaturated fat. Coconut milk is made up of 48 percent lauric, (the only other place you can find this amount is in mother's milk) 17 percent myristic, 9 percent palmitic, 8 percent caprilic, 7 percent capric, 6 percent oleic, and a small percentage of other fats. The caprilic and capric fats are used to make medium-chain triglycerides which are then used for energy that lowers cholesterol from fat metabolism, which creates half as much acid as sugar metabolism. Caprilic and capric fats are also anti-fungal, thus once again reducing acid which in turn reduces the need for increased cholesterol to bind to acid.

When whole unsweetened coconut milk or coconut oil is added to an otherwise standard American diet, there is no change in the serum cholesterol and some studies have shown a decrease in total cholesterol. For example, when an "average American" diet was studied with the addition of 2 to 3 times more myristic, 4.5 times more lauric and 1.2 times more palmitic, there was no increase in serum cholesterol levels, and in fact, the cholesterol levels fell approximately 3 percent, from 177.1 mg to 171.8 mg during a 22 week feeding trial.

In studies where unsweetened whole coconut oil was fed to Wistar rats, Hostmark et al (1980) compared the effects of diets containing 10 percent coconut fat and 10 percent sunflower oil on lipoprotein. Coconut oil feeding produced significantly lower levels of pre-beta lipoproteins (VLDL) and significantly higher alpha-lipoproteins (HDL) relative to sunflower oil feeding.

Awad (1981) compared the effects of diets containing 14 percent coconut oil, 14 percent safflower oil or a 5 percent "control" (mostly soybean) oil on accumulation of cholesterol in tissues in Wistar rats. The synthetic diets had 2 percent added corn oil with a total fat a 16 percent. Total tissue cholesterol accumulation for animals on the safflower diet was 6 times greater than animals fed the coconut oil, and twice that of the animals fed the control oil.

Finally, Kaunitz and Dayrit (1992) reviewed some epidemiological and experimental data regarding groups of people who regularly eat coconut. They noted that the available population studies show that dietary coconut oil does not lead to high serum cholesterol, nor to high coronary heart disease, mortality or morbidity.

According to all the research, you can feel confident in the health benefits of adding unsweetened, organic coconut water, milk and coconut oil to your diet. They are a great source of good fats, proteins and minerals that will help maintain or lower high blood sugars, lower cholesterol, inhibit an increase in biological transmutations like yeast, provide minerals for healthy bones and blood, and provide an excellent source of fuel for energy production. You can also use unsweetened coconut flakes in your soups, on salads or on fish to give that pleasurable coconut taste. Check out Shelley's Coconut Macadamia Salmon recipe on page 77 or the Super Soy Coconut pudding on page 114.

You can purchase extra virgin coconut oil from the Garden of Life by calling 800-622-8986 or through their website: www.gardenoflifeusa.com.

Onions and Garlic

Onion and garlic are two of the earliest known food medicines. They were used for hundreds of years for colds and catarrhal disorders, and to drive fermentations and impurities out of the body system. Onions and garlic contain a large amount of sulfur and are especially good as buffers of acid, thus helping to maintain the delicate pH balance of the body fluids.

Onion and garlic work to significantly lower blood sugar. The principal active ingredients are believed to be the allyl propyl disulphide (APDS) and dialyl disulphide oxide (allicin), although other constituents such as flavonoids may play a role as well.

Experimental and clinical evidence suggests that APDS lowers glucose levels by competing with insulin for insulin-inactivating sites in the liver. This results in an increase of free insulin. APDS administered in doses of 125 mg per kilogram to fasting humans was found to cause a marked fall in blood glucose levels, and an increase in serum insulin. Allicin doses of 100 mg per kilogram produced a similar effect.

In another study, onion extract was found to reduce blood sugar levels during oral and intravenous glucose tolerance. The affect improved as the dosage was increased; however, beneficial effects were observed even for low levels that were used in diets (e.g., 25 to 200 grams). The effects were similar in both raw and boiled onion extracts. Onions affect the hepatic metabolism of glucose and/or increase the release of insulin, and/or prevent insulin's destruction.

The additional benefit that comes from using garlic and onions is their positive cardiovascular effect. They are found to lower lipid levels, inhibit platelet aggregation and are antihypertensive. So, liberal use of onion and garlic are recommended.

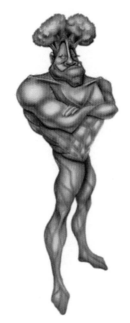

Doc Broc™ (Broccoli) is King of the Garden

Broccoli was grown in France and Italy in the 16th century, but was not well known in this country until 1923, when the D'Arrigo Brothers Company made a trial planting of Italian sprouting broccoli in California. A few crates of this were sent to Boston, and by 1925 the market was well-established. Since then, the demand for broccoli has been steadily on the increase.

Current scientific research that examines fresh broccoli and/or broccoli sprouts is being done at Johns Hopkins University. Data from animal studies suggests that a compound found in broccoli called glucoraphanin, a precursor to sulforaphane, boosts cell enzymes that protect against molecular damage from cancer-causing chemicals. Sulforaphane has been shown to mobilize, or induce, the body's natural cancer protection resources and help reduce the risk of malignancy.

Subsequent studies have found that sulforaphane could prevent the development of breast and colon cancer, as well as other tumors.

In my own research I have found that increased amounts of broccoli or broccoli sprouts act as a wonderful chelator of metabolic acid. They provide all the benefits of the cellular cleansing effects of chlorophyll and the compound of glucoraphanin, which acts as an anti-acid in the blood and tissues.

One of my favorite breakfasts is tomato, broccoli and avocado. I call it the true breakfast of champions!

Cucumbers

Cucumbers have been cultivated for thousands of years. Records indicate that they were used as food in ancient Egypt, and were a popular vegetable with the Greeks and Romans. The cucumber is one of the few vegetables mentioned in the Bible. It was probably introduced into other parts of Europe by the Romans and records of cucumber cultivation appear in France in the 9th century, England in the 14th century, and in North America by the mid-16th century.

Cucumbers are one of my favorite vegetables. I noticed that the more alkaline my diet became, the more I enjoyed the taste of cucumber. Its high water content, low sugar, and high potassium levels (433 mg per one medium-sized cucumber) makes this vegetable one of the best alkalizing agents for the blood and tissues that you can eat or drink. I always recommend to folks who are juicing to use cucumber instead of carrot for the base juice. The reason is because of the high sugar content of carrot juice.

Cucumbers are a cooling food, especially when used in fresh vegetable juices, or in a bath to draw acids out through the skin. When Dr. Young and I were in the West Indies we met a young boy who was suffering from elephantitis (see accompanying photo). He couldn't stop itching his skin. When he was put in a bath of cucumber water or a poultice of greens was applied to his skin the itching would immediately stop (itching is always from acid).

Cucumbers also contain several phytochemi-

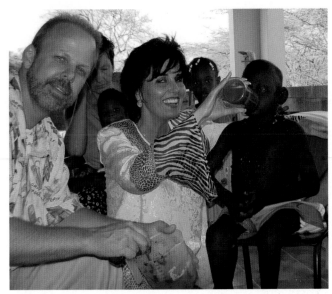

cals such as phytoesteroles which block the fermentation of the hormone estrogen. This in turn stops bacteria or yeast-producing acids that can be found in fat tissue, specifically the breast tissue, which may contribute to microcalcifications and breast or brain tumors. Cucumbers also contain monoterpenes which help to reduce gastrointestinal and metabolic acids, thus reducing the production of cholesterol to neutralize or bind to these acids.

Better Sources of Protein

Wheat Grass and Barley Grass

Have you ever wondered where the strongest animal in the world—the elephant—gets its strength? Do you have any idea how much animal meat an elephant eats? The answer is none. What about the cow or the horse–where do they get the protein to build their muscles? They get their protein the same way the elephant does—with their head to the ground. These strong animals do not count calories, they are not worried about balanced diet, and they are not concerned about how many grams of protein they are eating a day. They derive all their needed nutrients from grasses and leaves.

Why do I recommend drinking/eating grass?

The first reason is that grasses are some of the lowest calorie, lowest sugar, and most nutrient-rich foods on the planet. Consider the following information:

• Grasses have 25 percent more protein than meat, chicken, pork, turkey, fish and eggs
• Contains more than a hundred food elements
• More iron than spinach
• Contains every B vitamin, including B-12
• Rich in Vitamins E and K
• High concentration of laetrile, a compound used in natural cancer treatment
• A natural buffer of metabolic acids

The second reason is that grasses help to balance blood sugar levels. Drinking 3 ounces of juiced wheat or barley greens in one liter of distilled water in 15 minutes will help normalize high or low blood sugar.

Third, grasses are recommended because they contain chlorophyll. Chlorophyll is what gives a grass its green color; it is the "blood" of the plant. Interestingly, its molecular structure is similar to the hemoglobin of human blood. Hemoglobin is our body's oxygen transporter. A German chemist, Dr. Richard Willstatter, determined in 1913 that the two molecules closely resemble one another. He found that hemoglobin is composed of four elements: carbon, hydrogen, oxygen and nitrogen, organized around a single atom of iron. Chlorophyll has the same elements; however, they are organized around a single atom of magnesium. Chlorophyll is beneficial because it reduces the binding of carcinogens or acids to DNA in the liver and other organs. It also breaks down calcium oxalate stones for limitation.

Two of the best sources of chlorophyll are wheat grass and barley grass. Grass, this humble plant, is the doorway to health. Grasses have the power to regenerate our bodies at the molecular and cellular level. The Hebrew spelling for grass is "dalet, shin, aleph, deshe." Dalet translated means the lowest and the poorest—the door. Shin means birth, regeneration, coming forth. And aleph means the prime position, the letter of perfection. When we combine them all together we have the true meaning of the word grass–through the lowest of kingdoms on earth is the doorway through which we may be regenerated and come forth towards perfection of being. There it is, a message encoded in the Hebrew word for grass thousands of years before Dr. Willstatter described grass. The healing is in the grass, the greenness.

It has been said that "out of two or three witnesses shall every word be established." The Hebrew translation is the first witness, the second witness is the work of Dr. Richard Willstatter and there is a third witness.

The third witness is found in the ancient Chinese character for the word grass. This character has been found in the form of an oracle on bone fragments that date 2205 BC. What exactly is the picture for the word "grass?" It is two people kneeling at an altar, with arms upraised, petitioning the Heavens. Could this be Adam and Eve in the garden asking their creator what they should be eating?

There it is. The third witness. That Chinese character, thousands of years old, depicts our first parents "coming forth toward perfection of being" through the grass. It is an absolute match with the Hebrew characters.

A Fourth Witness for Truth

Another witness was found at Masada, written by the Essenes on what is known as the Dead Sea Scrolls. The Dead Sea Scrolls date back to the third century and are written in the Aramaic language. I quote from these ancient writings, "It is the angel of Life that flows through the blades of grass into the body of the son of Light, shaping him with her power. For the grass is Life and the Son of Light is Life, and Life flows between the Son of Light and the blades of grass, making a bridge to the Holy stream of light (the blood) which gave birth to all creation."

The answer is YES! Grass is the blood of life. I quote again from the Dead Sea Scrolls, "For if you crush within your hands the grass, you will feel the water of life, which is the blood of the Earthly Mother."

The molecular structure of the blood of grass is almost identical to our own blood. Is this by design? To drink the blood of the grass is to build our blood which heals and regenerates every cell in our body. The healing and regenerating power of grass is real—the power to regenerate our bodies at the cellular level, to heal and restore the perfect health and long life we were always meant to have! The truth has been hidden there in plain sight for thousands of years, in the most ancient languages, Hebrew, Chinese and Aramaic.

Sprouts

Sprouts are one of the very best foods on the planet. Sprouts are live plant foods that are biogenetic and life generating, which means they can transfer their vital life force energy to you. They are packed with plant compounds which aid digestion, contribute to cellular organization, and are alkaline forming. Sprouts can be grown in your kitchen from beans, lentils, grains, seeds, and almonds in any season, providing you with fresh organic produce when no other garden is available. They are easy to grow, some in as little as two days. Seeds for sprouting can be stored for long periods of time and can produce many times their weight in fresh produce that is full of vitamins, minerals, and complete proteins. They can be eaten alone, in salads, with grains, gently steamed with veggies as a snack, or sprinkled over soup. Everyone should store organic sprouting seeds and use sprouts in their daily diet.

One of the best types of sprouts to eat daily is soy sprouts. The soybean and soy sprout have been an ancient Chinese secret that we in the U.S. are just learning about. The soybean and its sprout are considered a complete food because they contain protein, carbohydrates and fat, as well as an impressive array of minerals. Soybeans and soy sprouts have the distinction of being the only vegetable source of complete protein, because they contain all eight essential amino acids. These amino acids cannot be produced by the body and must come from a dietary source. Soybeans and soy sprouts can supply us with even more protein than an equivalent amount of cheese, milk, eggs or even fish, and they contain no cholesterol or saturated fat. In other words, soybeans and soy sprouts are a high-quality vegetable protein which is better for us than beef, chicken, pork, turkey, lamb or eggs.

Soybeans and soy sprouts also contain calcium, phosphorus, iron, magnesium, thiamine, riboflavin, niacin, even B-12, and the essential fatty acids of both the Omega 3 and the Omega 6 oils, including lecithin.

There are quality soybean products such as edamame, tofu and powdered soy sprouts. If the soy sprouts are low-heat dehydrated at 88 degrees or less and then powdered, the concentration of proteins, fats and minerals is 20 to 30 times more than tofu or edamame. I strongly recommend including soybeans and especially soy sprouts in the diet because they contain many powerful and beneficial phytochemicals, namely:

Isoflavones, which the body converts into phytoestrogens, also known as plant estrogens. Phytoestrogens can help prevent the growth of hormone-dependent cancers. Dr. Neil Solomon, in his book *Soy Smart Health* states,

"Unlike synthetic hormone drugs, plants with estrogen-like substances appear to naturally support the female reproductive system. These substances make the plants useful for a number of disorders including breast, endometrial and prostate cancer prevention; menopausal and PMS miseries; and osteoporosis prevention. Phytoestrogens have the unique ability to compete with human estrogen for tissue receptor sites. In basic terms, this means that plant estrogens attached to the tissues where human estrogen normally would. Therefore, less human estrogen is able to attach to receptors. By introducing phytoestrogens to the body, we are able to decrease the activity of dangerous estrogens (like estradiol), while promoting a healthy balance of estrogen to progesterone in the body. Phytoestrogens also inhibit certain enzymatic reaction involving the growth of cancerous cells and boost bodies mechanisms that help to keep estrogen levels in check. These plants also contain an impressive array of other phytonutrients that provide powerful cellular protection,

especially against cancer."

Research studies reveal shocking differences in cancer rates between Asians living in Asia and their relatives in America. One study, which looked at breast cancer among Chinese-, Japanese- and Filipino-American women living in Los Angeles, San Francisco, Oahu, found that intake of soy was more than twice as high among Asian-American women born in Asia as compared with those born in the United States. Among immigrants, intake of soy decreased with years of residence in the United States. The study found that risk of breast cancer decreased when soy consumption increased in both pre-and post-menopausal women. The study points out the importance of daily soy consumption for continuing protection.

Daidzein, a special isoflavone found to inhibit the growth of cancer and to promote cell differentiation in animals. (Cancer cells are undifferentiated and functionless to the body.)

Genistein is the star isoflavone. It is an enzyme that can inhibit tumor growth and retard cancer development. Test tube and animal experiments have shown that genistein can block the growth of prostate cancer cells and breast cancer.

Protease inhibitors, which block the action of enzymes that may promote tumor growth. According to Ann R. Kennedy, Ph.D., a leading researcher at the University of Pennsylvania School of Medicine, protease inhibitors may be "universal anti-carcinogens" that work in many different animals to prevent or inhibit a wide range of cancers, from liver to colon to breast to pancreatic cancers. In my own research I have found protease inhibitors to be an excellent buffer or neutralizer of metabolic acids, thus protecting the pancreas and helping to maintain the delicate pH balance of the body fluids and blood sugar levels.

Phystic acid, a plant compound, which chelates or binds acids that promote cancer and the formation of tumors. Animal studies have shown that phystic acid can reduce the size and number of tumors in laboratory animals that were fed mycotoxins. (Mycotoxins are the acids from sugar fermentation by yeast and/or mold.)

Saponins, also found in chickpeas and in ginseng, have been shown in animal studies to lower the risk of certain cancers, including cancer of the breast, prostate, stomach, lung, and pancreas.

As you can see, the above phytochemicals can be of great benefit to our health and well-being. However, it is important to remember that fermented soy products, such as miso, tempeh, and soy sauce, should never be ingested. Especially avoid sauces like tamari, which is fermented with the fungus aspergillus flavus. Soy sauce was studied at the Cancer Center in the City of Hope Medical Center, Los Angeles, about 20 years ago. Researchers found it induced a number of cancers in animals. If you need something to taste salty, instead of fermented soy sauce, use Celtic or Real Salt, an alkalizing condiment that is healthful to the body.

Sodium Chloride/Celtic Salt (Real Salt™)—Essential for Good Health

An acidic body is at the root of pancreatic malfunction, sugar intolerance, insulin resistance and diabetes. Celtic sea salt is beneficial because it strongly alkalizes. It does this through biological transmutation where the sodium of the salt combines with nascent oxygen and becomes a new element, potassium. Proper pH balance will be replenished quickly through this process of changing sodium to potassium. Proper pH balance in the body in the body is achieved by maintaining a relatively high potassium content inside the cell and a correspondingly high sodium concentration in the fluids outside the cell. The concentration of salt diminishes in the blood as sodium biologically transmutates into potassium. In effect, we use up the salt in our diet in order to maintain the delicate pH balance of our bloodstream. Sodium or salt truly helps to maintain good health.

Public health policy should be guided only by proven facts. Current scientific research reveals that there are actually very few salt-related health problems. A healthy and active lifestyle demands a sufficient, though reasonable salt intake. The current medical dictate that our body can function on no salt at all or on a restricted ration of salt causes more problems than it tries to solve.

Life is closely dependent upon the presence of sodium. However, to clearly understand the role of sodium in biology, we should always view it along with the role of water and nascent oxygen, and the various ions of chloride, chlorite, potassium, calcium, magnesium, silica and hydrogen. That is why it is more important to study the co-activity of sodium with these other ions rather than the sodium element alone.

Sodium, in the form of sodium chloride, plays an important part in the primary processes of digestion and absorption. Salt activates the first enzyme in the mouth, salivary amalase. At this stage, sodium exposes food to the taste bud—one reason why food has always been salted "to taste." Salt also helps start digestion by breaking down food. In the parietal cells of the stomach wall, sodium chloride generates hydrochloric acid, one of the most important of all digestive secretions. If potassium is in excess in relationship to sodium, the body's enzyme pathway loses its ability to produce hydrochloric acid.

Most diets, especially the high protein and carbohydrate diets, require slightly more salt in order to prevent an excess of potassium over sodium. With salt present, the acidity of partially digested food is able to trigger off some needed natural sodium bicarbonate, derived from the supply of sodium chloride, as well as enzymatic and bile secretions from the gallbladder and pancreatic ducts. Without salt, no digestion is possible. In the many symptomologies of diabetes the requirement for an abundant supply of salt is vital for maintaining an adequate supply of sodium bicarbonate secreted by the pancreas. This sodium works to buffer acids coming out of the stomach and it biologically transmutates to potassium to maintain the delicate pH balance of the body fluids. It is no coincidence that your body is salted with sodium. The sodium ion from salt is a foundational element that is necessary for survival. Survival means maintaining the delicate pH balance of the blood and tissues. So eat liberal amounts of ocean salt (Real Salt™). The ocean contains all of the precious minerals our body requires for optimum function. This is the salt of life!

Fish

Another source of the precious minerals our body needs, as well as a source of the essential fats, is fresh fish (not farm-raised). Trout, salmon, mackerel, tuna, swordfish, sea bass, and other fresh water and ocean fish are high in heart-healthy omega 3 fatty acids. These essential fats help prevent clogged arteries and irregular heart-beats, ease depression, and appear to impede the inflammation involved in diseases such as diabetes. In fact, fish is the only food, aside from seaweed (which I also recommend strongly), that provides eicosapentaenoic acid (DPS) and docosahexaenoic acid (DHA), two important omega 3 fatty acids. A third fatty acid which fish also contains is alpha linolenic acid, or ALA.

Fish is an excellent low-acid source of all essential amino acids, several water-soluble vitamins of the B group, vitamins A and D, minerals including calcium, potassium, and trace minerals fluoride, iodine, zinc, and iron.

Getting your fish oils in a pill may be the best way to get all the omega 3s your body needs, especially if you just don't like fish. If you do like fish I would suggest two servings per week. If you don't, take a one-gram capsule of fish oil at least 3 times a day. Recently, an Italian study of more than 11,000 people found that those who took one gram of fish oil every day for three months had a 41 percent reduced risk of death from any cause compared to those taking the placebo, and the risk of sudden death from irregular heart beat dropped dramatically.

A Natural Sugar for Everyone, including Diabetics

There is one natural sugar and medicinal aid that has been used traditionally to treat diabetes. The plant is called Stevia Rebaudiana Bertoni, or

stevia, a plant native to Paraguay.

In 1931, a French chemist extracted a phytochemical called stevioside from the herb in the form of an intensely sweet, white, crystalline compound. The herb was then considered for use as a sweetener during the food shortages experienced by Britain during World War II. However, interest waned when sugar from cane and corn again became available.

Since that time, stevia has been used extensively in Central and South American countries, but the United States, Canada, and Europe have not embraced the herb as a sweetener, opting either for sugar from readily available sugar cane or sugar beet, or for aspartame-based and other artificial sweeteners as a sugar substitute.

More than 150 varieties of stevia exist, but Stevia Rebaudiana Bertoni is the only sweet stevia plant. Carbohydrate-based compounds from the stevia leaf can be isolated to glycosides known as steviosides. Stevioside is intensely sweet and is present at levels up to 13 percent in the leaves of Stevia rebaudiana Bertoni. Rebaudiosides and dulcosides are other sweet chemicals constituents of the plant that can be extracted.

Studies have found some positive effects and possible medicinal uses of stevia. The University of Illinois, *College of Dentistry Paper,* published in 1992, found that stevia is an intense and natural sweetener and is not carcinogenic, according to their data. A Japanese study from Nihon University, published in late 2002, revealed that the use of stevioside on skin tumors in mice inhibited the promoting effect of chemically induced inflammation.

A Taiwanese study showed the possibility of stevia's use for blood pressure regulation. A study undertaken on rats at Taipei Medical University and published in 2002 showed that stevioside lowered blood pressure. Another study done at Taipei Medical College, published in 2000, was undertaken on humans and concluded that "oral stevioside is a well-tolerated and effective modality that may be considered as an alternative or supplementary therapy for patients with hypertension."

Two recent studies by Jepson et al., from Aarhus University Hospital in Denmark, have found after test on rats and mice that stevioside should have potential in the treatment of Type-II diabetes. Natural therapists have been using stevia for many years to regulate blood sugar levels. According to a June 28, 2003, report on Australia's national broadcaster ABC (www.abc.net.au) the herb can be taken in droplet form with meals, bringing blood glucose levels to "near normal."

Users of stevia have also reported lower incidence of colds and flu. The herb can aid in weight-loss by reducing appetite and can be used to suppress tobacco and alcohol cravings. Stevia leaves also contain various vitamins and minerals including vitamin A, rutin, zinc, magnesium and iron.

Stevia has been used in South America for years as a treatment for diabetes. It has also been suggested that it can aid people to get off insulin. It has been used topically on skin cancers and to treat candidiasis.

In 1986, Brazilian researchers from the Universities of Maringa and Sao Paulo elevated the role of stevia in blood sugar (Curie, 1986). Sixteen healthy volunteers were given extracts of 5 g of stevia leaves every 6 hours for 3 days. The extracts of the leaves were prepared by immersing them in boiling water for 20 minutes. A glucose tolerance test was performed before and after the administration of the extract and the results were compared to another group that did not receive the stevia extracts. During a glucose tolerance test, patients were given a glass of water with glucose and their blood sugar levels were elevated over the next few hours. Those who had a predisposition to diabetes had a marked rise in blood sugar levels. The volunteers on stevia were found to have significantly lower blood sugar levels after ingestion of stevia. This is a positive indication that stevia can potentially be beneficial to diabetics in reducing blood sugars, as well as a sugar substitute in order to decrease a diabetic's sugar consumption for better blood sugar control.

Since 90 percent of Type II diabetics are overweight, stevia is an excellent non-calorie sweetener that can reduce caloric intake and thus contribute to weight loss due to excess acidity.

Shelley has included in the recipe section a wonderful green drink called the Avorado Kid Super Green Shake. This drink is sweetened with stevia and is an excellent alkalizer for the blood and tissues. My research indicates that the use of stevia does not increase blood sugar levels after ingestion. So enjoy Shelley's incredible recipes and some of the new Alkalarian desserts using stevia as a helpful supplement to reduce blood sugar levels.

All the Good Oils

I have previously discussed many of the wonderful oils or good fats and their medicinal benefits, but there is one more good fat that deserves consideration and should be included in your daily diet—cold pressed virgin olive oil.

Virgin Olive Oil

Virgin or cold pressed olive oil is a stable, health enhancing oil. It is an excellent source of monounsaturated fats and a rich source of unique components which can protect the microzymas of the genetic material from biological transmutation. It also provides beta carotene (pro-vitamin A) and tocopherol (vitamin E) which are excellent buffers of gastrointestinal and metabolic acids. Virgin olive oil contains 88 percent of its vitamin E in the form of alpha-tocopherol, which research has indicated protects the heart and arteries. These benefits are removed if the olive oil has been refined. So if it doesn't say virgin olive oil on the bottle then you now know it has been refined. If it is refined, remember that it has lost many if not most of its medicinal benefits.

Here is a list of some of the many beneficial health components of cold pressed virgin olive oil:

• Magnesium-rich chlorophyll to help in the formation of healthy red blood cells.
• Squalene, a precursor to phytoesterols which helps reduce acidity.
• Phytoesterols (in the form of beta-sitosterol) which protect against cholesterol absorption.
• Triterpenic reduces inflammation due to acidity.
• Caffeic and gallic stimulate the flow of bile

which helps to alkalize food coming out of the stomach, reducing stress on the pancreas.

• Phenolic compounds protect against fermentation of fats and cholesterol creating more acid. 2-phylethanol stimulates the production of fat-digesting enzymes in the pancreas.

• Triterpenic found only in olive oil stimulates pancreatic digestive enzymes to alkalize food coming out of the stomach.

• Cycloartenol lowers the amount of circulating cholesterol and increases the bile excretion to help remove acidity and increase alkalinity of the food coming out of the stomach.

For all of these reasons I suggest using liberal amounts of olive oil with salads, vegetable stir-fry or in soups. One or two tablespoons a day can go along way to maintaining the delicate alkaline pH balance of your blood and tissues.

CHAPTER 1

Foundation

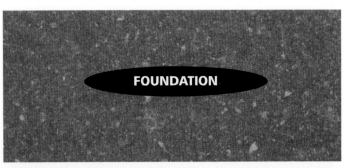

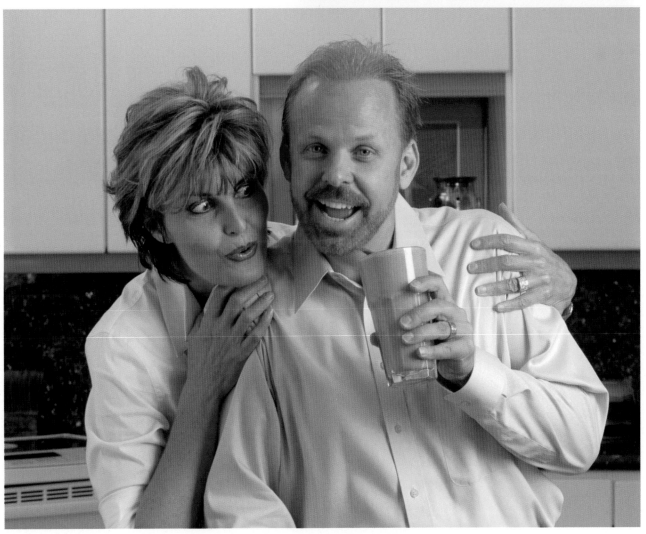

The Raw Perfection Morning Monster Juice

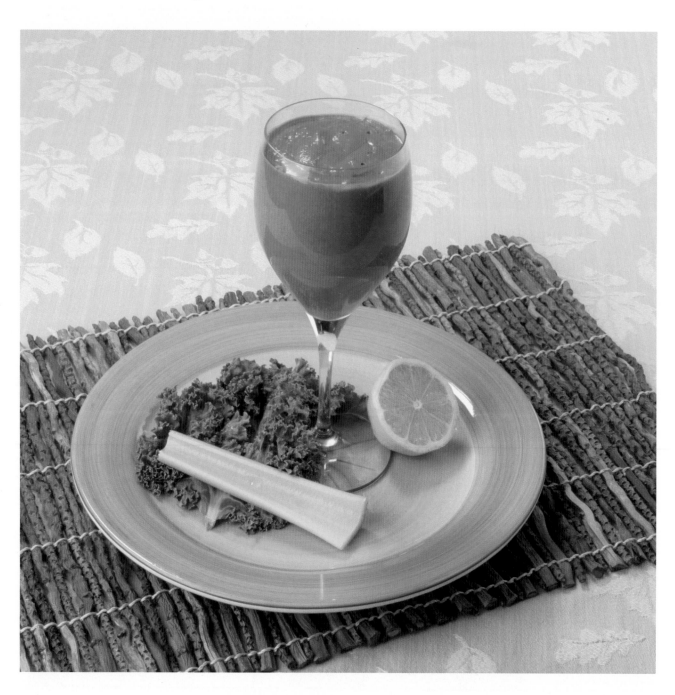

The Raw Perfection Morning Monster Juice.

By Mike Nash. Serves 1–2.

This juice is great when you need something that's going to stick with you until mid-day; the fat will help you feel full. Besides providing that fat, the avocado is the key to the creaminess of this smoothie.

1 bunch of kale

1 whole head of celery

1 lemon

1 handful of spinach leaves

1 avocado

1 teaspoon green powder

1 chili pepper

Put kale, celery and lemon through juicer, then combine in blender with remaining ingredients.

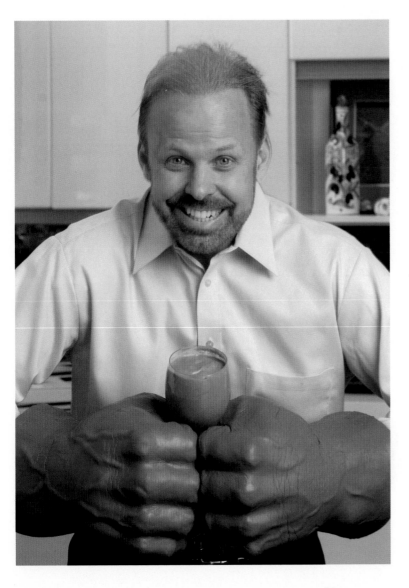

"And to every beast of the earth, and to every fowl of the air, and to ev ery thing that creepeth upon the earth, wherein there is life, I have given every green herb for food: and it was so."

Genesis 1:30

The AvoRado Kid Super Green Shake

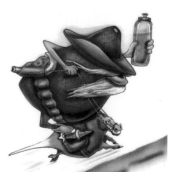

The AvoRado Kid

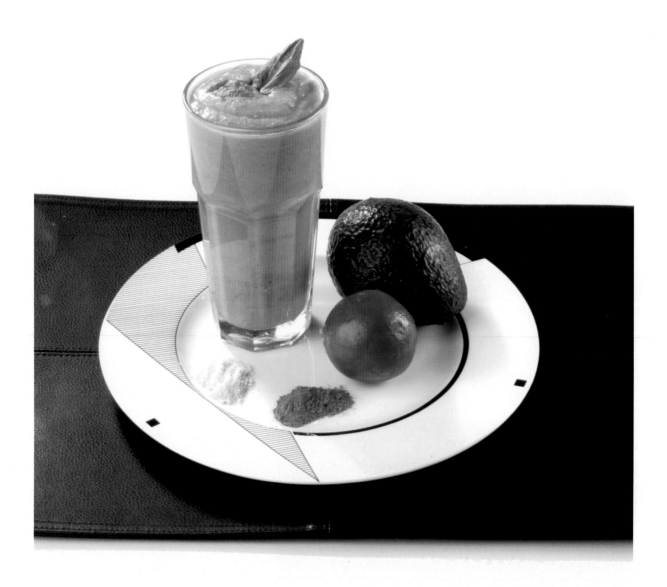

AvoRado Kid Super Green Shake

This is by far our favorite cool green shake, and we've enjoyed it for breakfast, lunch and dinner—or anytime we want a snack. It's a great way to get the concentrated nutrition and chlorophyll of green powder and soy sprouts powder (and an especially great way to get it into your kids). The cucumber and lime cool the body, and the essential fats in the avocado and soy sprouts make this shake one that you can burn on for many hours. Serves 1.

Blend on high speed to a thick, smooth consistency. Serve immediately.

Variations:

* Add 1 teaspoon of almond butter for a nuttier flavor.
* Add coconut milk or fresh almond milk for a creamier shake.
* Make a parfait by layering the shake with layers of dehydrated unsweetened coconut and sprinkle some of the coconut on top.
* Substitute a grapefruit or lemon for the lime for a different taste.
* Add 1 tablespoon fresh grated ginger.
* Add some seasonings that are bottled in oil (without alcohol) for a new exciting twist of flavor.
* In the summer, freeze AvoRado Kid into pops for a cool frozen treat. You can also completely freeze and then partially thaw small portions of the shake, then chop it up to enjoy as a slush.

1 avocado
1/2 English cucumber
1 tomatillo
1 lime (peeled)
2 cups fresh spinach
2 scoops soy sprouts powder
1 scoop of green powder
1 pkg. stevia (I use Sweet Leaf with Fiber)
6–8 ice cubes

"It has been said, 'Never trust a skinny chef' but I say, Always trust a skinny chef . . . she'll keep you out of the hospital!"

Shelley Redford Young

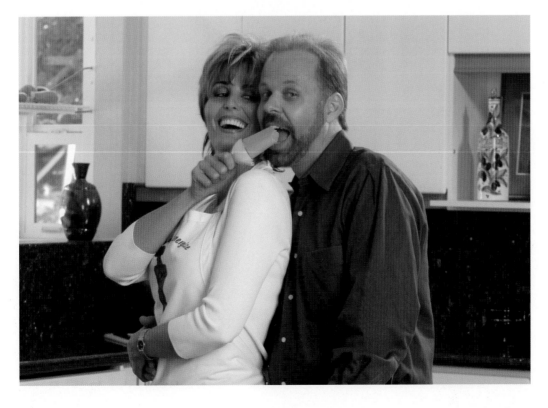

Fresh Silky Almond Milk

Serves 4–6; makes approximately 1 quart.

4 cups of fresh raw almonds
Pure water
nylon stocking (for straining)

Soak 4 cups of fresh raw almonds over night in a bowl of water. Drain. Place the almonds into a blender until it is one-third full (about two cups), then add pure water to fill the blender up. Blend on high speed until you have a white, creamy looking milk. Take a nylon stocking—I use a (clean!) white knee-high nylon stocking—and pour the mixture through it over a bowl or pan, and let it drain. Squeeze with your hand to get the last of the milk through the nylon. Thin the milk with water to desired consistency. Drink as is, or add a bit of stevia to sweeten it. Use in soups, shakes or puddings. Almond milk will stay fresh for about 3 days in the refrigerator. Serves 4–6 (makes approximately 1 quart).

Note: Use the solids you strained out with the stocking in the shower for a great body scrub!

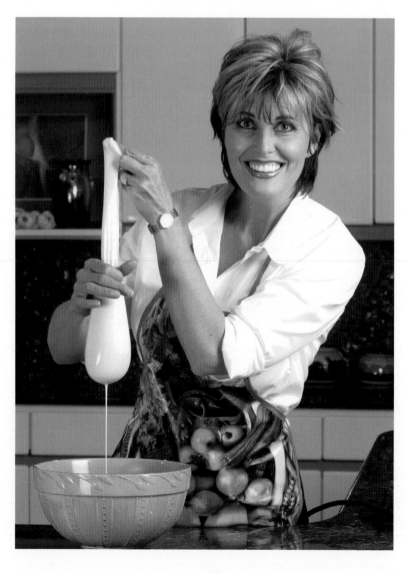

Fresh Silky Almond Milk

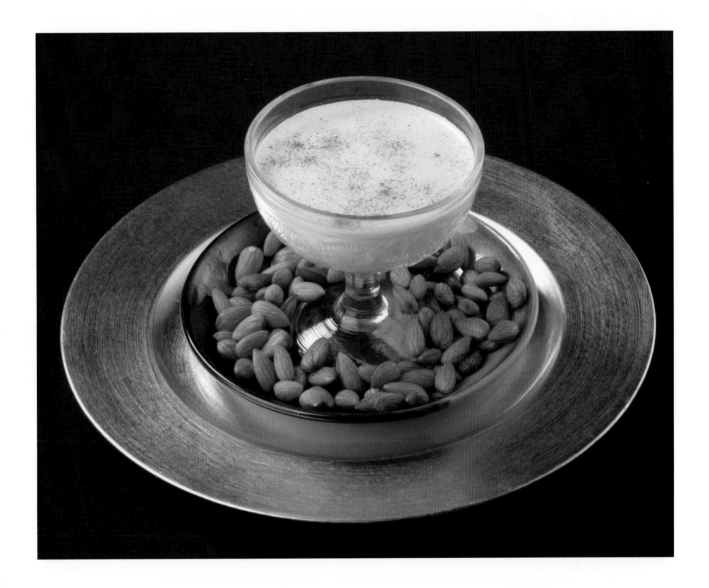

"I no longer feel like I'm stuck in the kitchen... I feel like I'm painting edible masterpieces with God's healing palette!"

Shelley Redford Young

Very Veggie Shake

By Parvin Moshiri. Serves 1–2.

1 cup distilled water

1/4 cup flax seed oil or olive oil

2 small cucumbers, sliced

1 cup spinach

2 avocados

1/3 head Romaine lettuce

1/2 cup broccoli

1/4 cup cilantro

1/4 cup parsley

2 stalks of celery, cut into pieces

1/8 cup fresh mint leaves (or 1 teaspoon dry)

2 medium limes (or 1 lemon)

1/8 cup fresh dill (optional)

Place water in a blender then add oil. Turn blender on low speed and add remaining ingredients one at a time. When everything is chopped up, turn up blender to high speed until you get a beautiful smooth and creamy green shake.

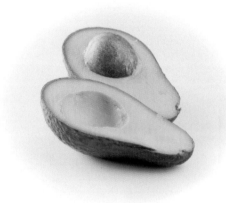

Minty Mock Malt

By Matthew and Ashley Rose Lisonbee. Serves 2.

1/2 English cucumber

juice of 1 lime

juice of 1 grapefruit

1 avocado

1 cup raw spinach

1/2 can coconut milk

1 teaspoon green powder

2 teaspoons soy sprouts powder

8–10 drops pH drops

2–4 sprigs for fresh mint leaves or 1/2 teaspoon mint flavoring (no alcohol)

14 ice cubes

Combine all ingredients and blend to desired consistency.

Variation: Leave out the ice cubes, and freeze malt into pops.

Clean and Simple Soup

By Eric Prouty. 2nd place, Alkalarian recipes, the pH Miracle Recipe Contest. Serves 1–2.

Place ingredients in food processor with S blade. Mix until almost smooth. Serve garnished with mint leaf.

1 cucumber, cubed
1 avocado, cubed
mint (optional)

Romaine Peppered Salad

By Randy Wakefield. Serves 6.

Combine garlic and oil in a small bowl; let stand 30 minutes. Add the minced onion, tomato, and jalapeno; stir well and set aside. Lay down whole romaine leaves to cover 6 salad plates. Tear endive and remaining romaine into small pieces and layer over top. Lay pepper strips on top. Drizzle each serving with 1 1/2 tablespoons of the oil mixture. Spray with Bragg Liquid Aminos or Real Salt to taste.

1 clove minced or pressed garlic
2 teaspoons cold pressed olive oil or Essential Balance Oil
2 teaspoons minced onion
2 teaspoons tomato finely chopped
1 small jalapeno pepper, seeded and finely chopped
3 cups romaine lettuce
3 cups Belgian endive
1 red bell pepper, cut into strips
1 yellow bell pepper, cut into strips
Bragg Liquid Aminos/Real Salt, to taste

Moroccan Cole Slaw

By Eric Prouty. 2nd place, pH Miracle Recipe Contest. Serves 4–6.

Shred cabbage in food processor with shredder wheel. Mix all ingredients well in a bowl. Let sit for at least half an hour before serving to allow flavors to blend and seeds to soften.

1/2 head green cabbage
1/2 head red cabbage
1/3 cup fresh lemon juice
1 1/2 teaspoons Chinese 5 Spice powder
1 teaspoon caraway seeds
4 tablespoons olive oil

Soothing Cooling Tomato Soup

The combination of fresh tomatoes and avocado makes this silky smooth cooling soup high in lycopene and lucene. Serves 2.

6 medium tomatoes, juiced and strained (pour through a fine mesh strainer or a nylon knee-high stocking)

1/2 avocado

3/4 cup fresh coconut water (make sure this is fresh, taken from a coconut)

1 cucumber, juiced

Real Salt to taste

stevia (optional)

Blend until smooth. For a sweeter soup, add stevia to taste.

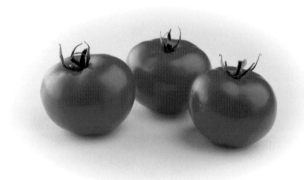

Cool Raw Red Soup

This is a raw soup made by juicing all your veggies and then blending them with avocado and some fresh coconut water. The soup has a cooling effect, and is light and refreshing—perfect for a hot summer day. Serves 2–4.

1 beet

1/2 large English cucumber

4 stalks celery

1–2 carrots

1 small clove garlic

1/4 cup fresh cilantro

1/2 avocado

1/4 cup fresh coconut water (which should be clear and slightly sweet)

grated veggies (for garnish)

Juice first six ingredients, then pour juice through a clean knee-high nylon stocking or a fine wire mesh strainer. Mix in blender with avocado and coconut water. Garnish if desired with grated veggies.

Soothing Cooling Tomato Soup

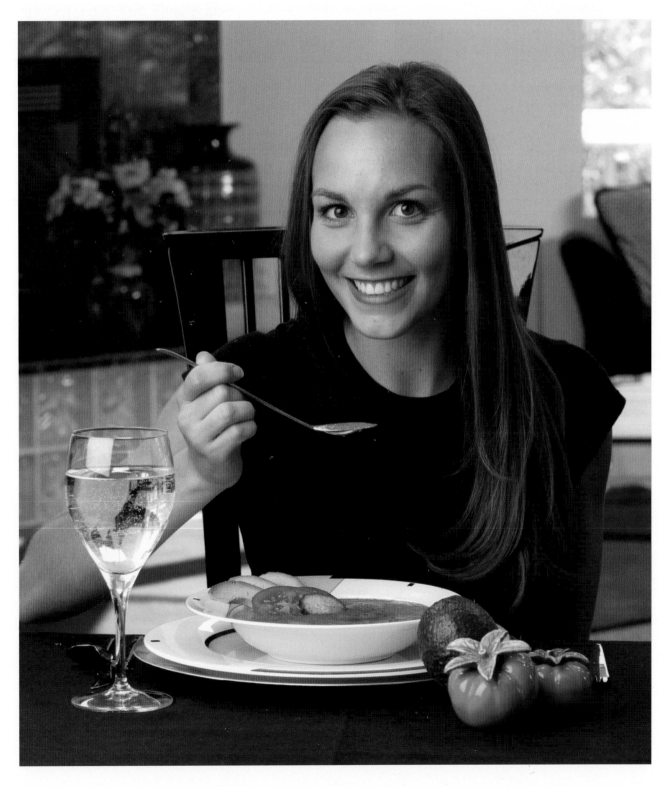

Green Gazpacho Two Ways

By Eric Prouty. 2nd place, the pH Miracle Recipe Contest. You can prepare this soup simply for a refreshing taste, or you can make it robust with the addition of herbs (which is what my family prefers). Either way, it's a wonderfully alkaline soup, packed with chlorophyll. Serves 4–6.

2 avocados
2 green bell peppers
6 roma tomatoes
1 1/2 large English cucumbers (or 2 average size)
1 head Romaine lettuce
1/2 red onion
3 cloves garlic
1/4 cup fresh lemon juice
1/4 teaspoon Real Salt
2 tablespoons olive oil
1 1/2 teaspoons basil
1/2 teaspoon dill
1/4 teaspoon oregano
1/8 teaspoon sage powder

Chop all vegetables. Mix avocado, lemon juice and garlic in food processor (with S blade), until smooth and empty into bowl. Process tomatoes and romaine until smooth, and add to bowl. Pulse peppers, cucumbers and onion until chunky (approximately 1/8–1/4 inch) and empty into bowl. Mix well with salt and olive oil, and herbs if desired.

French Gourmet Purée

By Eric Prouty. 2nd place, pH Miracle Recipe Contest. This is a beautiful soothing alkaline puree. Sometimes I like to double the amount of lettuce to thin it out a bit. Serves 6.

1 avocado
2 stalks celery
1 head Romaine lettuce
1 small tomato
1 handful spinach
1 small cucumber, peeled
2 cloves garlic
1/3 onion
2 tablespoons olive oil
Herbes de Provence
sprouts (optional)

Purée all vegetables with a Green Star/Green Power juicer with a blank blade for puréeing, doing the onion last. Mix in olive oil, and Herbes de Provence to taste. Serve with sprouts sprinkled on top.

Green Gazpacho Two Ways

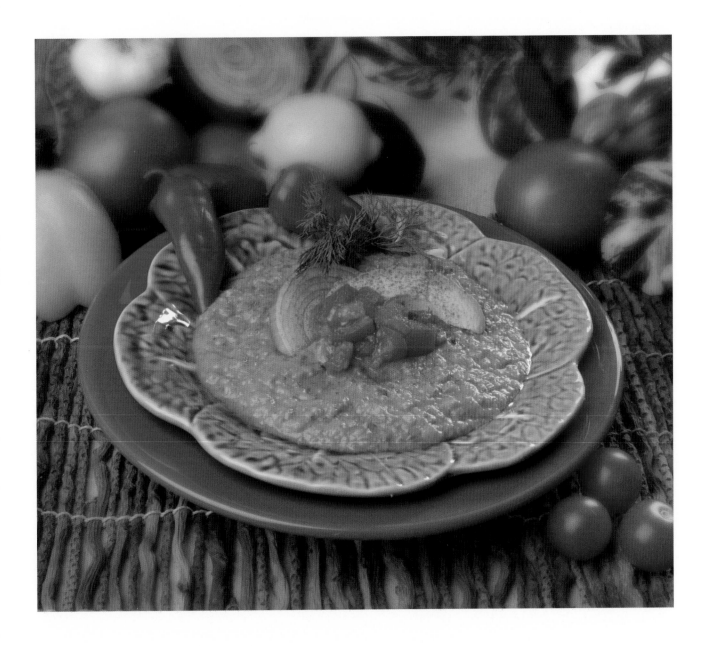

Moroccan Mint Salad

By Lisa El-Kerdi. Best in Show, pH Miracle Recipe Contest. The perfect accompaniment to North African Bean Stew (p. 84). Serves 4–6.

2 cucumbers, seeded and minced by hand

4–6 scallions, minced by hand

1 bunch parsley, stems removed

1 bunch mint, stems removed

1/2–1 jalapeno

4 tomatoes, seeded and finely chopped

1/2 cup lemon juice

1/4 cup olive oil

1/2 teaspoon Real Salt

1/2 teaspoon paprika

Mince herbs and jalapeno in food processor, or by hand. Mix in bowl with cucumbers and scallions. Add tomatoes. Stir in lemon juice, olive oil and spices. Sahateck! (To your health!)

Refreshing Grapefruit Salad

By Kathleen C. Waite. I like to arrange the avocado slices in this recipe like flower petals, and put the grapefruit mixture inside as the center of the flower. Serves 2–4.

1 tablespoon flax oil

1 tablespoon Bragg Liquid Aminos (or Real Salt or Herbamare, to taste)

1–2 teaspoon sesame seeds

1 teaspoon Mexican Seasoning (Spice Hunter) (optional)

1 grapefruit peeled and cut into bite size pieces

1 cup chopped celery

1 red bell pepper, chopped or thinly sliced

1 cup jicama, grated

1 handful of fresh cilantro

1 avocado, peeled and sliced lengthwise

1/4 –1/2 cup soaked almonds, chopped

Combine first four ingredients (through Mexican Seasoning) to make dressing. Combine remaining ingredients except avocado and almonds in a bowl and toss with dressing. Arrange on a plate with avocado slices. Top with almonds.

Moroccan Mint Salad

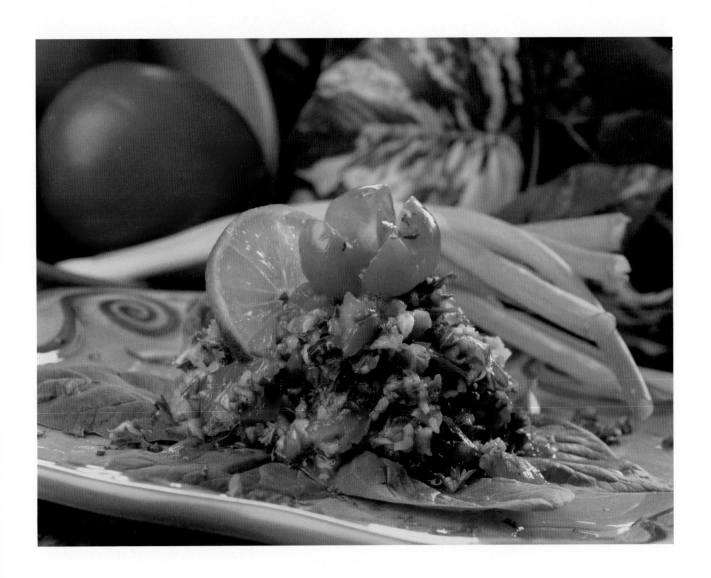

Alkalarian Cole Slaw

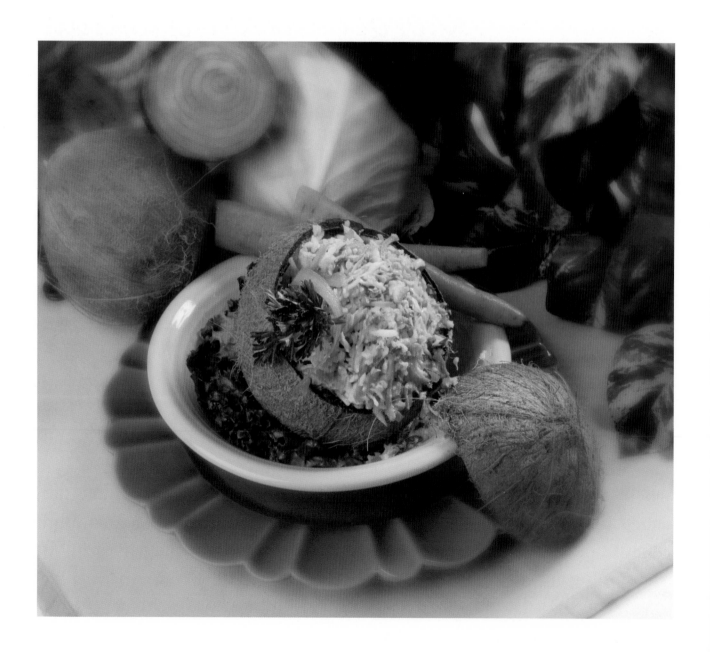

Alkalarian Cole Slaw

By Sheila Mack. 3rd place, The PH Miracle Recipe Contest. Serves 4–6.

Toss the first four ingredients (through parsley) in a bowl. Blend coconut milk and arrowroot (if needed to thicken) in blender. Blend in remaining ingredients and toss with cabbage mixture. This tastes best if you let it sit and chill for awhile before serving, to give the flavors a chance to blend.

1/2 head green cabbage, shredded

2 medium carrots, shredded

1/2 small red onion, sliced thinly into strips

1/2 cup chopped Italian parsley

1 cup coconut milk (make it fresh by blending the coconut water and meat of a coconut in a blender)

1 teaspoon arrowroot powder (optional)

1/2 teaspoon sea salt or to taste

1/4 teaspoon celery seed

1/2 tablespoon fresh lime juice

2 tablespoons grapeseed oil

dash of cayenne pepper

stevia (optional)

Flaxseed Oil and Lemon Dressing

By Roxy Boelz. 3rd place, pH Miracle Recipe Contest. Serves 2–4.

Combine basil and garlic in blender. Add the rest of the ingredients and blend to desired consistency.

1/2 cup lemon juice

1/4 cup flaxseed oil or Udo's oil

1/4 cup water

1/3 bunch, fresh basil (or 1–2 teaspoons dried)

2 cloves of garlic

1/4 cup olive oil

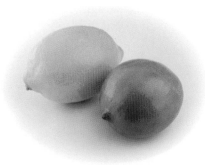

Avocado Grapefruit Dressing

By Debra Jenkins. 1st place for best transitional recipes, in the pH Miracle Recipe Contest. Serves 1–2.

1 large avocado
juice of 1 small (or 1/2 large) grapefruit
stevia (optional)

Blend in blender, then add stevia to balance tang, if desired.

Avocado Salad Dressing

By Gerry Johnson. Delicious over a garden salad. Serves 4–6.

2 ripe avocados, peeled
1 cup freshly juiced celery juice
Seasonings (optional)

Mix together in a blender, adjusting amount of juice to achieve desired consistency. Add whatever seasonings appeal to you—or enjoy as is.

Scrap Soup

By Mary Seibt. Serves 4.

3 large carrots
2 celery stalks
4 stalks asparagus, chopped
1 large yellow onion
6 cups of distilled water
4 teaspoon of instant vegetable broth (yeast free)
1 1/2 teaspoon cumin
2 teaspoons dill
Real Salt, to taste
2 teaspoons The Zip or 21 Spice Salute

Shred carrots and celery in food processor. Bring water to boil, adding vegetable broth and onion. Once boiling, turn off the heat. Add carrots, celery, stalks of asparagus and let stand until vegetables are tender. Cool enough to put in blender and mix all ingredients. Serve warm.

Rustic Guacamole

By Maraline Krey. 2nd place in transitional recipes, in the pH Miracle Recipe Contest. This rustic guacamole can be served as a side dish, as a main course salad over baby spinach drenched in lime juice and avocado or olive oil. For a great salsa to use over fish, add a cut up grapefruit. Serves 4–6.

Combine in a large bowl and toss as you would a salad. Keeps in the refrigerator for two days.

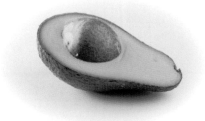

- 4 Haas avocados, diced into 1/2–3/4 inch cubes
- 1/2 bunch cilantro, cut up (use kitchen scissors)
- 1 extra large tomato (or 2–3 small ones), diced
- 1/4 onion, chopped
- juice of 2 or 3 limes
- 1/2 teaspoon Real Salt
- 1/2–1 teaspoon The Zip (Spice Hunter) or hot sauce (optional)

Fresh Garlic Herb Dressing

Serves 4.

Blend all ingredients in a food processor or blender until well blended.

- 3/4 cup Essential Balance Oil (a blend of organic flax, pumpkin and sunflower oils from Omega Nutrition)
- juice of one large lime
- 1 teaspoon Italian Pizza Seasoning (Spice Hunter)
- 2–3 cloves fresh garlic, minced
- 1/2 teaspoon onion salt (Real Salt puts out a nice blend)
- 1/2 teaspoon Vegetable Rub (Spice Hunter)
- 1/4 teaspoon fresh minced rosemary
- 1/4 teaspoon Heat Wave Seasoning (very hot spice from The Cape Herb and Spice Company)

"And there were some who died with fevers, which at some seasons of the year were very frequent in the land—but not so much so with fevers, because of the excellent qualities of the many plants and roots which God had prepared to remove the cause of diseases, to which men were subject by the nature of the climate."

Alma 46:40
Book of Mormon

3 Citrus Dressing

This is a nice thick dressing with a sweet and sour taste . . . very zingy! It is good when you are phasing out Thousand Island and other sweet dressings. Makes about 2 cups; serves 6–8.

juice of 1/2 large pink grapefruit

juice of 1 lime

juice of 1 lemon

1/2 teaspoon chicory root powder (try Nature's Taste by Amazon) OR 6–10 drops of liquid stevia or 1 package stevia (I use Sweet Leaf brand with fiber)

extract or 1–2 packets of powdered Stevia.

1 teaspoon hot mustard powder

4 tablespoons dried onion

2 teaspoons garlic powder

2 teaspoons dried basil

1/4 teaspoon dried rosemary

1/2 teaspoon Real Salt

pinch of Zip

1 1/2 cups Essential Balance Oil (Arrowhead Mills or Omega Nutrition brand) or other healthy oil

1 heaping tablespoon flaxseeds

Put all but last two ingredients into a food processor or blender and blend well. With machine still running, add oil, then flaxseeds, and let machine run until all ingredients are well emulsified.

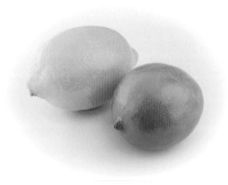

Citrus Flax and Poppy Seed Dressing

By Derry Bresee. Serves 4.

1/2 cup carrot juice

1/2 cup freshly squeezed citrus juice (juice of 2 lemons and 1/2 grapefruit is about 1/2 cup)

1/2 teaspoon dry powdered mustard

2 tablespoons minced dry onion

1 teaspoon flaxseeds (optional)

1 teaspoon minced fresh garlic

1 teaspoon basil

1/2 teaspoon salt

1 tablespoon poppyseeds

1 cup flaxseed oil

Combine all but the last two ingredients in a blender and blend, using the flaxseeds if you want a thicker dressing. Add poppyseeds and pulse briefly. With blender on low, slowly pour oil in until dressing is emulsified and thickened.

Flaxseed Oil Dressing

By Derry Bresee. Serves 2–4.

Blend in blender. Serve immediately, or refrigerate until use.

Variation: Use your favorite herbs or spices instead of the seasonings listed here.

- juice of 1 lemon or lime, about 1/4 cup
- 1/2 teaspoon onion powder
- 1/2 teaspoon garlic powder
- 1/2 teaspoon salt
- 1/2 teaspoon chopped dry basil
- 1 tablespoon flaxseeds (optional—use if you want to thicken the dressing enough that it spreads like mayonnaise)
- 1/2 cup flaxseed oil (or enough to be twice as much as the juice)

Creamy Tomato Soup

By Dr. Gladys Stenen. Serves 2.

Liquefy in blender. Heat just to warm.

- 4 Roma tomatoes (or equivalent)
- 2 green onion tips (about 1 inch of white/light green part)
- 1/4 green pepper
- 1 cup vegetable broth
- 1 avocado or 1/4 soft tofu package (if you use tofu, this would be a Framework recipe)
- 1 teaspoon sea salt
- pepper to taste

Tera's Hearty Party

By Tera Prestwich. Serves 4–6.

1 head of broccoli

1 head of cauliflower

1 red bell pepper

1 green bell pepper

1 orange bell pepper

2 stalks of celery (sliced)

1 bag of edamame (soy beans), shelled

3 green onions

1/2 clove of minced garlic

1/4 cup of Bragg Liquid Aminos or 1–2 teaspoons Real Salt

1/2 cup Essential Balance oil (or oil of choice)

1 tablespoon Garlic Herb Bread Seasonings (Spice Hunter)

Chop broccoli, cauliflower, celery, green onions and bell peppers. Mix together. Cook edamame as directed and add to mix. Then add in the essential oil, minced garlic, Bragg Liquid Aminos, and Garlic Herb Bread Seasonings. Toss together and garnish with Zip.

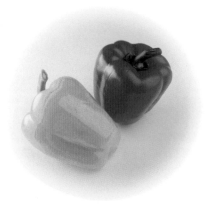

Fantastic Kale

By Wendy J. Pauluk. Kale is a calcium rich chewy dark green leafy vegetable. It is good juiced or in the raw salad below. Serves 4.

1 bunch kale

1/4 cup olive oil

1 small red onion

1 red bell pepper

juice of 1 lemon

Zip seasoning, to taste

Tear kale into bite-sized pieces. Do not use center stem. Slice red onion and red bell pepper into thin strips and add to kale. Add olive oil and toss. (You may add more or less depending on size.) Refrigerate overnight in covered bowl. Add juice of 1 lemon and Zip seasoning before serving.

Chi's Green Drink

By Jill Butler from her friend, Chi. Serves 2.

Blend in blender until smooth.

1 head Romaine or Boston lettuce (use the greenest leafy parts, omitting the really light green stems if you wish)

3 cloves of garlic

1 lemon

3/4 cup water

1/2 cup olive oil

1 piece of cut fresh ginger (optional)

dash of sea salt

dash of cayenne pepper

Add a combination of all or one or none of the following:

2–4 basil leaves, or to taste

1/4 cup parsley, or to taste

1/8–1/4 cup watercress (leaves only), or to taste

1 cucumber, peeled

1/2–1 cup steamed broccoli

(Or use whatever combination of green veggies you like. Experiment!)

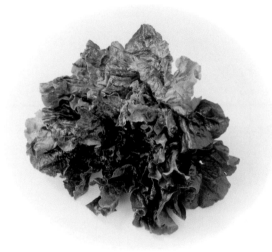

Paul's Breakfast in a Blender.

By Paul A. Repicky, Ph.D. This is a chewy sort of breakfast (or anytime) shake which will keep you going for hours. Serves 1.

Mix all ingredients in blender on medium speed (or higher if you like it smoother). Adjust quantities to taste. This recipe usually makes 32–34 ounces.

1/2 large non-sweet grapefruit (or 1 small one), outer layer of rind peeled off (the white inner rind is quite nutritious) and core and seeds removed

1 handful of sprouts (alfalfa, or clover, or other)

1 handful of fresh spinach

1/3 cup fresh ground flax seed

1–2 tablespoons Udo's oil

2 cups broccoli, chopped

1/2 cup cucumber, chopped

1 1/2 cups water

Spicy Kale Slaw

By Deborah Johnson. 2nd place for Alkalarian recipes, in The pH Miracle Recipe Contest. Serves 4.

1 ripe avocado, seeded and peeled

1 cup jicama, peeled and cubed

juice of 1 lime

1 scoop soy sprouts powder

1 tablespoon Udo's oil

1/2 teaspoon Real Salt or to taste

Place all of the above in a food processor or VitaMix and blend until smooth, stop machine. While above ingredients are still in processing bowl, add the following in order given:

1 carrot, washed and cut into 1 inch pieces

the spine of three leaves of kale, cut into 1 inch pieces

1/2 to 1 jalapeno pepper (depending how hot you like your food)

1 tomatillo, peeled and quartered

1/2 teaspoon mustard seeds

3 leaves kale (with spine removed and cut into 1 inch pieces, add with carrot layer) torn into large pieces.

Process, just until all ingredients are chopped to desired consistency. If using a processor pulse and scrape bowl. If using a Vita Mix use tamping tool, do not over process. This is a good lunch for one or a great side dish for two.

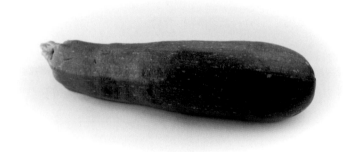

Creamy Watercress Soup

By Deborah Johnson. Serves 4–6.

1 head cauliflower (cut into 1-inch pieces)

2 cups pure water

2 cups vegetable broth

2 cups fresh watercress, chopped (reserve a sprig or two for garnish)

1 cup zucchini pieces

1 cup broccoli pieces

1 cup celery pieces

4 green onions, tops removed

1/4 cup extra virgin olive oil

Real Salt to taste

Boil water, remove from heat, add cauliflower and allow to rest for 5 minutes. Place cauliflower and water in food processor or blender and process until smooth. Add vegetable broth and remaining ingredients and blend until desired consistency is reached. Do not over blend. Serve warm or chilled. Garnish with a sprig of watercress.

"If you want to see a miracle . . . grow a garden!"
Shelley Redford Young

Spicy Kale Slaw

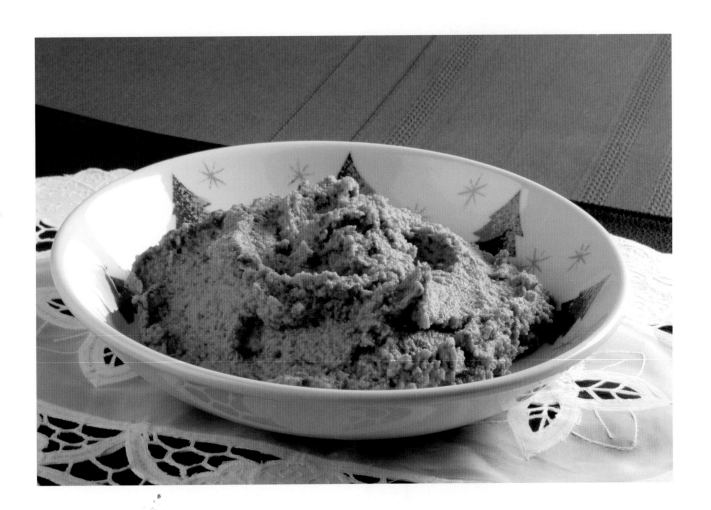

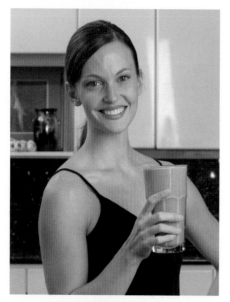

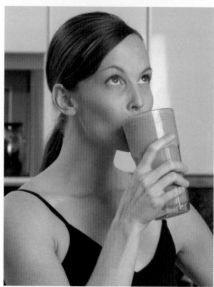

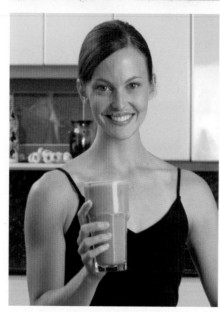

Got Greens?

CHAPTER 2

Framework

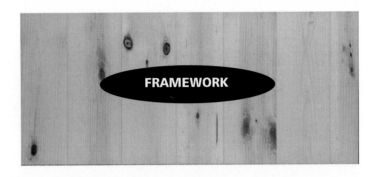

"May all be fed. May all be healed. May all be loved."

John Robbins
from *Diet for a New World*

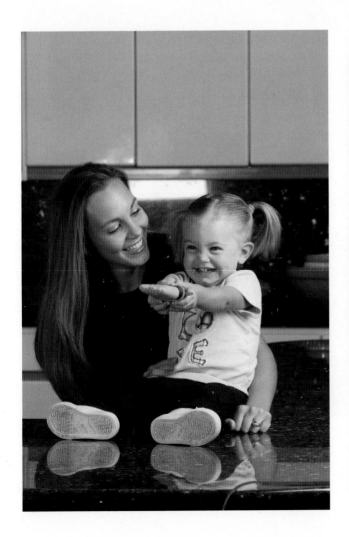

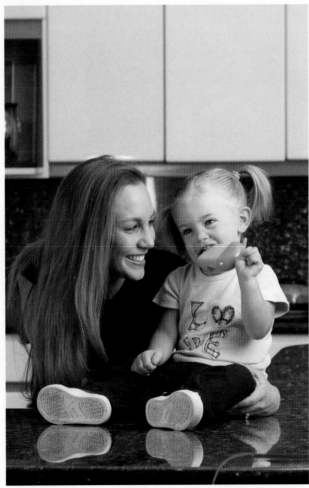

Carrot Crunch

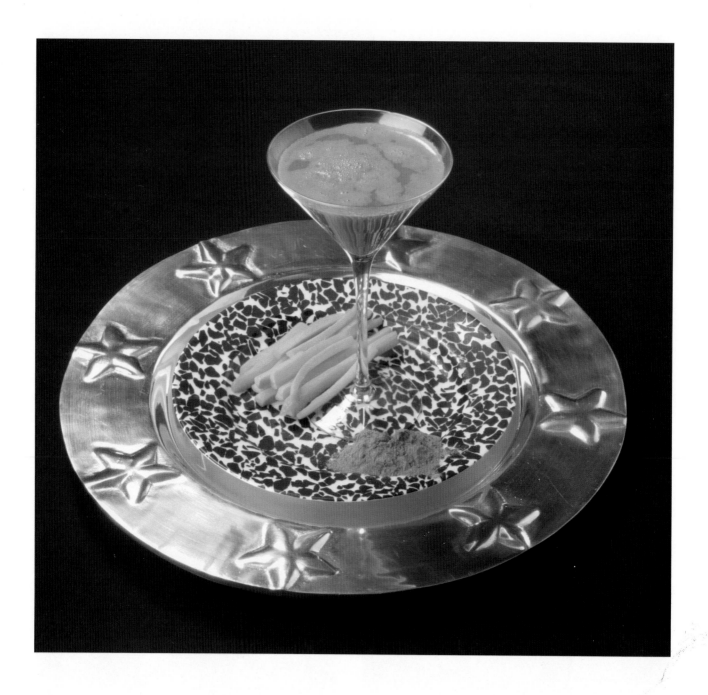

Zesty Lemon Ginger Shake

By Karen Rose. Serves 1.

Mix all ingredients together in the blender until creamy. Add Rice Dream, almond milk or water if necessary for desired consistency.

Variation:
To make this shake higher in protein, as well as even more lemony, add:
1 lemon or lime
1–2 teaspoons soy sprouts powder
1 teaspoon green powder
2 teaspoons stevia (with fiber)
1/4 cup soft tofu
6–8 ice cubes

1 lemon, peeled and chopped
2 tablespoons chopped fresh ginger
1 avocado
1 small cucumber
1–2 teaspoons soft tofu

Carrot Crunch

By Randy Wakefield. Serves 1.

Combine ingredients in electric or hand blender and blend until smooth. Serve sprinkled with nutmeg.

1/2 teaspoon green powder
7 drops of pH drops
1 cup fresh carrot juice
1 chopped carrot
4 ice cubes

Mary Jane's Super Simple Spaghetti

By Mary Jane Medlock. Serves 2.

Cut spaghetti squash in half (clean out seeds). In a baking dish put spaghetti squash (facing down) in a 375 degree oven. Bake for approximately 45 minutes or until done. Let cool for about 5 minutes. Using fork, scoop out the spaghetti squash into a bowl. Add the remaining ingredients and toss. Eat warm or cold.

1 medium spaghetti squash
2 medium ripe vine tomatoes chopped
juice of one small lemon
1–2 cloves of fresh garlic minced or chopped
2–3 tablespoons of olive oil
fresh ground pepper
1/4 teaspoon of oregano

Navy Bean Soup

By Roxy Boelz. 3rd Place, pH Miracle Recipe Contest. Serves 4–6.

1 cup aduki beans, soaked overnight

1 cup navy beans, soaked overnight

1 small onion, chopped

2 large carrots, grated

Real Salt to taste

2 teaspoons fresh ginger, grated

1 cup celery, chopped

nutmeg or cardamom

Cook the beans till just tender. Cool slightly. If necessary, add water to get the consistency of soup you want. Add the salt, onion, carrots and ginger. Transfer to a food processor or blender and process to the texture desired. You can add celery with the ingredients to be blended, or afterwards for crunchiness. Serve sprinkled with nutmeg or cardamom or a spice of your choice.

Tortilla Soup

By Cheri Freeman. 3rd place, pH Miracle Recipe Contest, transitional. Some people like to use organic chicken broth instead of veggie. This soup, minus the tortillas and tofu, would be great for a liquid feast. Serves 4–6.

3 cups yeast-free vegetable broth (read the label—Morga and Pacific brands have no yeast in them)

1 cup pureed fresh tomatoes or packaged strained tomatoes (with no preservatives or additives)

8 oz. baked seasoned tofu, sliced or coarsely chopped

2–3 teaspoons olive oil

2 tablespoons garlic, chopped

2 jalapenos, seeded and very finely chopped

1/2 cup cilantro, very finely chopped

1/2 onion, very finely chopped

Real Salt to taste

garlic pepper blend to taste

1 avocado, diced

sprouted grain tortillas (1/2 for each serving) (optional)

Preheat oven to 200 degrees. Place your tortillas directly on the baking rack until they are crisp, about 10–20 minutes. Pour your broth and tomato puree in a saucepan and begin heating on very low heat while preparing vegetables and tofu. In a small skillet, brown tofu in olive oil. Add to broth. Add garlic and spices. When warmed, turn off heat, and add avocado to soup. Serve topped with broken bits of tortilla sprinkled on top for some added crunch.

Vegan Chili

By Cheri Freeman. 3rd place, pH Miracle Recipe Contest, transitional foods. Great on cold nights! Serves 2–4.

In a saucepan or cast iron pot, brown crumbled patties in olive oil. Add all remaining ingredients except salad. Adjust seasonings to your own taste. If you don't like it too hot, you can seed your jalapeno. Put about half the chili in a blender, add salad mix, and puree. Pour back into the remaining chili and stir thoroughly. Serve topped with vegan cheese.

2 soy veggie burger patties, crumbled (Boca brand is good)

1/4 cup olive oil

1/2 onion, chopped

1 jalapeno, chopped (with or without seeds, depending on how hot you want it)

1 tablespoon chili powder

1 teaspoon Real Salt

2 cloves garlic, chopped

3 cups strained tomatoes

2 cups tossed salad (mixed greens, chopped red and yellow peppers, chopped carrots, etc.)

vegan cheese shreds (optional)

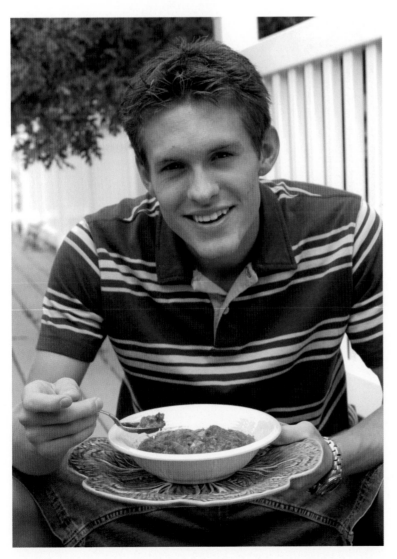

Roasted Leek Ginger Soup

This is one of Shelley's favorite soups! Serves 4.

In a soup pot, stir-fry leeks and ginger in oil until softened and browned on edges. Pulse chop leek and ginger in food processor and return to soup pot. Add almond milk, broth and Real Salt. Warm and serve.

Variation: Add garlic with the leeks and ginger, and stir in diced roasted bell peppers.

1–2 tablespoons olive or grapeseed oil

1 cup fresh almond milk (see recipe, p. 36)

1 leek, thoroughly cleaned and sliced in 1/3-inch slices

1 teaspoon fresh ginger, thinly sliced

1/2 –1 teaspoon Real Salt

2 cups vegetable broth

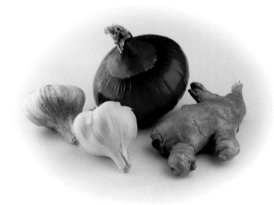

Spicy Latin Lentil Soup

By Cathy Galvis. Serves 4.

2 cups lentils

6 cups water

2 carrots, sliced

1 celery stalk, chopped

1/2 green pepper, chopped

1/2 red bell pepper, chopped

1 onion chopped

2 cloves garlic, minced

2 bay leaves

1 teaspoon Bragg Liquid Aminos

1 teaspoon olive oil

1/2 teaspoon jalapeno pepper, seeded and chopped

1/4 teaspoon cayenne pepper

1/8 teaspoon black pepper

1/4 cup cilantro, chopped

In a large pot, add the water and lentils and bring to a boil. Add the carrots, cayenne pepper, black pepper, Bragg Liquid Aminos and bay leaves. Return to a simmer and cover. In a separate pan, sauté the onions, garlic, green and red peppers, celery and jalapeno pepper in the olive oil for a few minutes. Set aside. Cook the lentils for approximately 20 minutes and add the sautéed onions and peppers. Cook for 10 more minutes or until the lentils are soft. Serve garnished with the cilantro.

Roasted Leek Ginger Soup

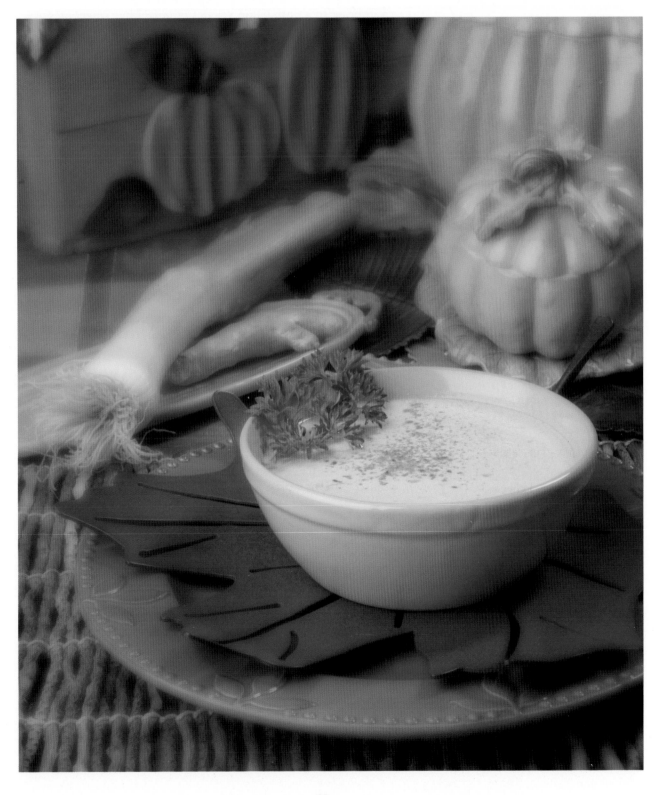

Tera's Any Meal Veggie Soup

By Tera Prestwich. Serves 6.

1 medium onion
3 cloves of garlic (1teaspoon minced)
5–7 sun-dried tomatoes
2–3 tablespoons Bragg Liquid Aminos
1 tablespoon parsley (1/4 cup fresh)
2 teaspoons real salt
pepper, to taste (I use 1 teaspoon)
1 quart vegetable broth
1 quart water
1 head cauliflower
1 bunch broccoli
1 bunch celery (I use the leaf also)
1 pound carrots
1/2 pound fresh green beans
1/2 pound peas

Blend first seven ingredients (through pepper) in food processor. Put in soup pot and cook until onion is clear. Add broth and water and bring to a boil. Chop veggies (and feel free to get creative with any veggies here, instead of or in addition to the ingredients above), and add to the soup. Add more water if necessary. Cook until veggies are just tender but still a little crunchy.

Celery Root Soup

Celery Root (or celeriac) is the bulb root of the celery stalk. It a large, gnarly, rough skinned root. Not the most attractive of vegetables sitting in the produce section, but none the less, delicious and very good for you. Serves 4.

1–2 tablespoons grapeseed oil
1 large celery root, peeled and chopped into
    large bite-sized chunks
2 white onions, chopped
1 cup water or vegetable broth
Real Salt, to taste

Wash celery root thoroughly with a brush to loosen dirt trapped in the gnarls. It is somewhat difficult to peel, so break out a good sharp knife or trusty peeler.

Sauté onions in oil until softened and lightly browned. Add celery root and water and steam for 5–10 minutes until veggies are done. Put soup in blender with enough water or broth to cover the top of the onion and celery root. Blend until smooth and creamy. Add more water if necessary to reach desired consistency. Season to taste with Real Salt. Serve warm as a soup, or spoon over veggies as a sauce or gravy. Experiment with adding your favorite seasonings.

Veggie Almond Chowder

This soup is even better the next day after it has stored in the refrigerator overnight and the flavors have blended.
Serves 4.

Put first eleven ingredients (through curry paste) in a blender and blend until very smooth. Place in soup pot. Steam or steam fry the veggies, and add to soup pot. Warm and serve.

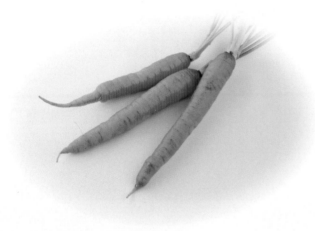

3 cups soaked almonds (blanch to remove skins if desired) OR 2–4 cups fresh almond milk (see recipe on p. 36)

juice of 1–2 lemons

1 garlic clove

1 teaspoon Garlic Herb Bread Seasoning (Spice Hunter)

1 quart vegetable broth (I use Pacific Brand)

2 teaspoons dehydrated tomato powder (The Spice House)

1 teaspoon real salt

1/2 teaspoon cumin

1/2 teaspoon celery salt

black pepper or The Zip to taste (Spice Hunter)

1/4 teaspoon green Thai curry paste

1 head broccoli

1 yellow onion

2–3 stalks celery

1/2 pound of fresh green peas from the pod

Creamy Curry Broccoli Soup

By Dr. Gladys Stenen. Serves 2.

Liquefy in blender, then warm.

2 cups broccoli

2 cups vegetable broth (adjust amount to reach desired thickness)

1/4 soft tofu package (or more to taste)

1 teaspoon curry powder

salt and pepper, to taste

Creamy Cauliflower Confetti

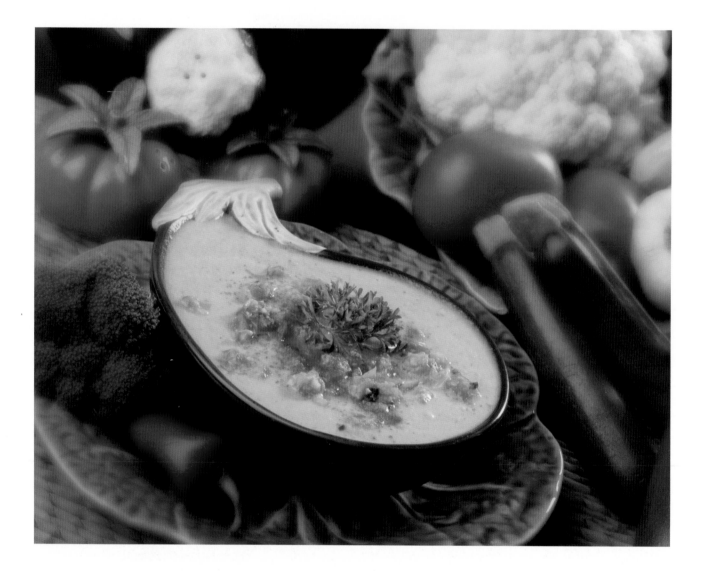

"There is only one sickness, one disease, and one treatment: The overacidification of the blood and tissues due to an inverted way of living, eating, and thinking."

Dr. Robert O. Young

Creamy Cauliflower Confetti Soup

This soup is deceptively creamy—you'd think it had dairy in it. The roasted veggie bits give it, its confetti appearance. Sprinkle roasted bell peppers over the top and a dash of The Zip for more color. Serves 2–4.

Preheat oven to broil. Cut the veggies into bite-size pieces. Place on non-stick cookie sheets and rub with grapeseed oil. Broil until lightly browned, 10–20 minutes. While veggies are roasting, make almond milk and place in soup pot. When veggies are done, add cauliflower to the blender with half the onion and half the celery root and blend with enough of the almond milk to get a rich and creamy consistency. Place mixture in soup pot. Pulse chop the remaining veggies in a food processor until minced and add to soup. Stir to separate the bits. Add broth and stir well.

1 head of cauliflower

3 yellow crookneck squash

4 zucchini

2 yellow onions

2 pkg. cherry tomatoes

1/2 celery root

8 cloves garlic

1 quart fresh almond milk
  (see recipe on p. 36)

1 quart vegetable broth

1/4 –1/2 cup grapeseed oil

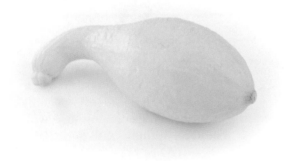

Special Celery Soup

This is a perfect soup for an appetizer before your main course, or on a day when you're tired and need to give your mind, body, and digestive tract, a rest. Serves 4–6.

Sauté celery, leek and ginger in oil until softened. Place half in the blender with half the almond milk and blend well. Mix with remaining veggies and almond milk and warm. Thin with vegetable broth if desired.

1 tablespoon coconut oil

1 whole head of celery, including core and
  leaves, sliced

1 leek (sliced white part)

1 tablespoon ginger, grated

1 quart fresh almond milk
  (see recipe on p. 36)

vegetable broth (optional)

Lentil-Brazil Nut Salad

By Roxy Boelz. 3rd place, pH Miracle Recipe Contest. Serves 1–2.

1 1/2 cups lentils, cooked
1 cup edamame beans, shelled
1/4 cup lime juice
dash of Real Salt
1/2–1 teaspoon fresh ginger
1 cup spinach, rinsed and chopped
2–3 tablespoons chopped Brazil nuts
sprinkle of parsley

Combine the lentils, edamame beans, and spinach. Combine the lime juice, salt and ginger, and stir into bean mixture. Sprinkle with Brazil nuts and parsley.

Lemony Green Bean Salad

By Roxy Boelz. 3rd place, pH Miracle recipe contest. Serves 1–2.

1 cup green beans, cut
1 cup zucchini, sliced
juice of 1 lemon
1/2 cup daikon radish, sliced and chopped
1/2 cup dulse flakes
1/2 cup parsley, chopped

Lightly steam the green beans. Cool. Combine with zucchini and daikon. Stir in lemon juice. Sprinkle with dulse flakes and parsley.

Jerusalem Salad

By Sue Mount. Serves 4.

1/3 cup tahini
2 tablespoons olive oil
1–2 cloves garlic, crushed
juice of 1/2 lemon
3 tablespoons parsley
Real Salt, to taste
1 cucumber, diced
6 Roma tomatoes, or 3 regular tomatoes, diced

Mix first six ingredients thoroughly in a salad bowl to make a dressing; add water to thin if necessary. Add cucumber and tomatoes and toss. You can let this sit for an hour to allow flavors to meld.

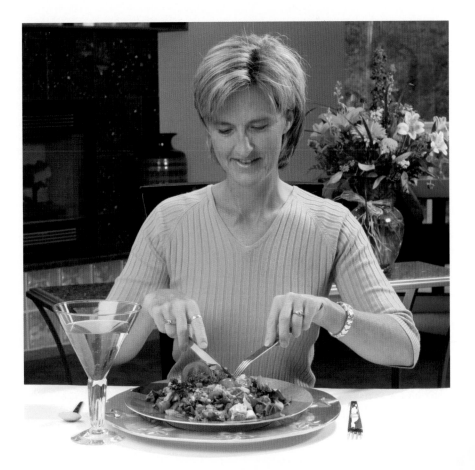

"Let your food be your medicine and your medicine be your food."

Hippocrates

Popeye Salmon Salad

By Maraline Krey. 2nd place, pH Miracle Recipe Contest. This salad would also be delicious without the fish! To get the most juice out of them, roll the lemon and limes on the counter before cutting and squeezing them. Serves 4.

Place salmon in a glass baking dish. Marinate in water and juice of lemon and one lime for two hours, turning over after an hour. Preheat oven to 400 degrees. Bake salmon in the liquid for 25 minutes, then place under the broiler for 5 minutes to brown the top. Make dressing by combining the remaining lime juice, oil, pepper, salt, seeds and pine nuts. Use kitchen scissors to cut spinach and basil leaves into bite-sized pieces. Add into a large salad bowl with whichever of the diced vegetables you choose. Toss with dressing and let sit until salmon is ready. To serve, cover dinner plates with salad, and top with pieces of salmon.

Rustic Guacamole (p. 49) makes an excellent accompaniment.

1 1/2 lb. salmon fillet (cold water preferred)
juice of 1 lemon
juice of 3 limes, divided
4 oz. water
2 oz. avocado oil or extra virgin olive oil
Real Salt
ground pepper
1 oz. ground flax seed
1 oz. poppy seed
handful of pine nuts (optional)
1 lb. spinach leaves
1/2 cup of basil leaves
1 cup hearts of palm, diced
1 cup diced carrots (optional)
1 cup diced celery (optional)
1 cup diced tomato (optional)
1 cup diced asparagus (optional)

Quinoa Salad

By Charlene Gamble. Quinoa is a versatile grain. Small and lacy, it makes a good substitute for rice. Serves 4.

1/2 cup quinoa
1 cup vegetable broth
1 teaspoon cumin, divided
1/2 cup brown rice
1 cup water
1 15 oz. can black beans, drained, rinsed and drained again
1 1/2 red peppers, finely diced
1/3 cup minced cilantro
1 1/2 bunches green onion, chopped
2 celery sticks, chopped
4 tablespoons fresh lime juice
3 tablespoons olive oil (or whatever healthy oil you prefer)
Real Salt to taste

In a small saucepan, combine rice, water and half of cumin. Bring to a boil, cover, reduce heat and simmer 35 minutes. Rinse quinoa in sieve. In another small saucepan, combine with broth and half of cumin. Bring to a boil, cover, reduce heat and simmer 15–20 minutes. Combine cooled grains in a bowl with remaining ingredients. Refrigerate for awhile before serving to blend flavors.

Potato Vegetable Soup

By Terry Douglas. This is a nice full bodied veggie soup. Serves 4.

4–6 small red potatoes
1–2 tablespoons olive oil
1 medium yellow onion, chopped
2 cloves garlic, chopped
2 cans vegetable stock
1 celery, sliced
2 carrots, sliced into rounds
salt, pepper and cayenne, to taste
1–2 cups baby spinach leaves
1/2-inch fresh ginger, sliced or julienned
a few leaves of cilantro
1/2 cucumber, chopped
1 tomato, chopped
1/2 green or red pepper, chopped
Bragg Liquid Aminos (optional)
basil (optional)

Cook potatoes in boiling water until tender (about 20 minutes). In a separate soup pan, over low heat, sauté onion in olive oil; add garlic when the onion is almost done. Add broth, celery and carrots. If you don't have lots of liquid, add a can of water. Heat until warm, 3–5 minutes. Veggies should still be crunchy. Season to taste with salt, pepper and cayenne. Remove from heat. Add spinach and ginger. To serve, quarter potatoes, and divide into soup bowls.

Optional: Add a drop of Bragg Liquid Aminos and a basil leaf in each bowl. Add soup, and top with cilantro, cucumber, tomatoes and pepper. Serve immediately, with crackers or sliced avocado.

Steamed Beets with Greens

By Kathleen Waite. Serves 2–4.

Cut beet head from greens and scrub well. Trim ends and cut into quarters or halves, depending on the size of the beet. Steam in steaming basket on high for 10 minutes and remove from heat. Meanwhile wash and rinse beet greens. Fold them over a couple of times and cut into pieces. When the beets are done, place the greens over the beets in the basket, put the lid back on, and let stand for 5 minutes to soften the greens. Meanwhile, combine lemon juice, oil, and Bragg Liquid Aminos or salt. Put greens and beets into a serving bowl and stir with dressing. Top with almonds.

1 bunch fresh beets with greens attached
1/2 juiced lemon
1 tablespoon flax oil
1 tablespoon Bragg Liquid Aminos (or Real Salt or Herbamare, to taste)
1/4 –1/2 cup almonds, soaked and chopped (optional)

Asparagus with Garlic-Lemon Sauce

By Roxy Boelz. 3rd place for alkalizing recipes, in The pH Miracle Recipe Contest. Serves 1–2.

Lightly steam asparagus. Add lemon juice, garlic and ground flaxseed and stir. Serve warm or cold.

2 cups asparagus, steamed
1/3 cup fresh lemon juice
3 tablespoons ground golden flaxseed
1 garlic clove, chopped

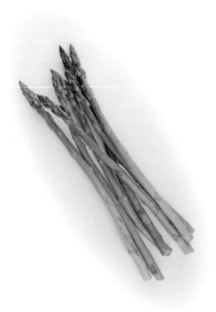

Sunshine Dressing

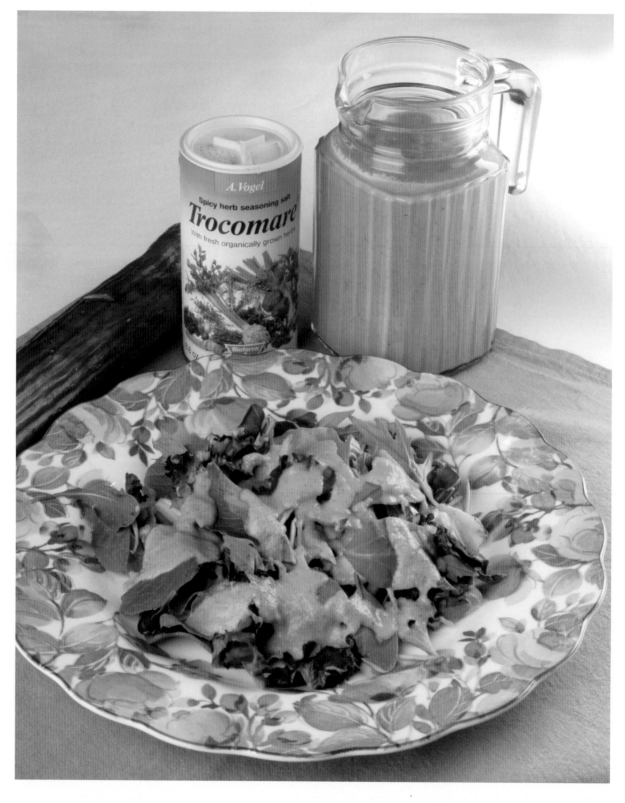

Sunshine Salad

By Frances Parkton. 2nd place, in the pH Miracle Recipe Contest. Serves 6–8.

Combine all ingredients except dressing in serving bowl, and serve topped with dressing.

2 cups cooked quinoa

1 cup minced zucchini

2 cups minced broccoli

1 cup minced onion

1 red or orange bell pepper, minced

1 cup pine nuts

2 tablespoons toasted sesame oil

salt, to taste

tomatoes, chopped, to taste

parsley, minced, to taste

1 recipe Sunshine Dressing (see below)

Sunshine Dressing

By Frances Parkton. 2nd place, in the pH Miracle Recipe Contest. This is a great versatile dressing, dip, or sauce. Somewhat like an all around Hollandaise Sauce that you could use for most any dish. Great over tacos or burritos too! Serves 6–8.

Put all ingredients in VitaMix or blender and blend to make salad dressing. Adjust seasonings to taste.

Variation: Add 1 cup cherry tomatoes for a wonderful gazpacho.

2 cups minced cucumber

2 sun-dried tomatoes

1 cup onions, minced

4 jalapenos, minced

1 cup green bell pepper, minced

1/2 cup olive oil

1/2 cup avocado oil

1/4 cup Vegannaise (make sure it doesn't have vinegar)

2 teaspoons Mexican Seasoning (Spice Hunter)

juice of 2 limes

2 teaspoons Herbamare

1/2 teaspoon cayenne pepper

2 teaspoon fresh garlic

Almond Butter Dressing

By Debra Jenkins. 1st place, Transitional Recipes, in the pH Miracle Recipe Contest. Serves 2–4.

1–2 tablespoons almond butter

1/4 pound soft tofu

1 fresh clove garlic

2–4 tablespoons oil (Udo's blend, Essential Oil blend, or olive oil)

juice of 1 lime

1/2–1 tablespoon Bragg Liquid Aminos

1 teaspoon Mesquite Seasoning (Spice Hunter)

1/2 teaspoon onion powder

Blend ingredients together.

Almond Avocado Dressing

By Debra Jenkins. 1st place, Best Transitional recipes in the pH Miracle Recipe Contest. Serves 2–4.

2 tablespoons raw almond butter

1 clove garlic

1/2 medium avocado

1 tablespoon fresh lemon juice

1 tablespoon Bragg Liquid Aminos

3 tablespoons Essential Oil Blend

3 tablespoons Udo's oil (or favorite olive oil)

dash of garlic powder

1/4 teaspoon onion powder

1/2 teaspoon Frontier Spice Fajita Seasonings

Blend in blender until smooth and creamy. Chill.

Variation: Add 3–4 sun dried tomatoes

More Peas Please

By Dianne Ellsworth

Mix the first nine ingredients (through lemon zest) in a salad bowl. Make a dressing by mixing the remaining ingredients together thoroughly. Pour half of the dressing over the vegetable mixture and toss well. Add more dressing to taste.

4 oz. pea pods, washed, trimmed and cut into bite-sized pieces

4 oz. pea shoots, 4-inches long cut in half (or pea sprouts 2-inches long)

10 oz. frozen baby peas thawed

1/2 small red onion, sliced thinly into 1/4 inch strips

2 cloves garlic, finely minced

3/4 cup raw pumpkin seeds

2 tablespoons fresh baby dill weed

2 tablespoons freshly grated ginger

zest of 1/2 lemon

juice of 1 lemon

3 tablespoons olive oil

2 tablespoons grapeseed oil

1 tablespoon Udo's oil

1/2 teaspoon dried dill weed

1/2 teaspoon Garlic Herb Bread Seasoning (Spice Hunter)

Bragg Liquid Aminos, to taste

Texas Style Guacamole

By Amy Efeney. Serve chilled or at room temperature, with veggies or tortilla chips (try Shelley's homemade tortilla chips with Mexican Seasoning in The pH Miracle*). This is a great after work pick-me-up snack. Serves 2.*

Mash all ingredients together with a fork for chunky guacamole, or use a blender (a new one might have a "salsa" setting) or food processor for smoother texture.

2 large avocados

1 whole jalapeno pepper (more or less)

1/2 habanero pepper (or not—they're really hot!)

1/4 cup onion

1/4 cup roasted (or fresh) tomatoes

1 teaspoon fresh lemon juice

1 dash garlic powder

1 dash Real Salt

1 dash fresh ground pepper

Pesto Dressing/Sauce

Serve cold over salad or veggies or legumes. Serves 4.

1/2 jar Garlic Galore Pesto (Rising Sun Farms brand, has no dairy)

1/2 cup olive oil (cold-pressed virgin)

2–3 sun dried tomatoes

1 teaspoon Garlic Herb Bread Seasoning (Spice Hunter)

1/2 cup raw macadamia nuts

Put all ingredients into a food processor and process until smooth, adding water to desired consistency.

RANCHadamia Super Sauce

This is a great way to get off of dairy ranch salad dressing. It is also great as a dip for raw veggies, or as a spread in wraps. Macadamias are rich in unsaturated fats, and contain calcium, magnesium, and many of the amino acids that make complete proteins. Serves 6–8.

2 cups of fresh raw macadamia nuts

juice of 1 lemon

2–6 teaspoons of LiteHouse Salad Herbs seasoning (a freeze-dried combination of parsley, shallots, chives, onions and garlic)

6–9 sun-dried tomatoes

1 1/2 teaspoons Cafe Sole Lemon Pepper (a blend of lemon, pepper, onion, and sea salt from Spice Hunter)

2 squirts of Bragg Liquid Aminos

water

With food processor running (using an S-blade), add all ingredients except water through the top shoot. Start with 2 teaspoons of seasoning, then taste and adjust the amount. Mix well and then slowly pour in a large glass of water in until you reach desired consistency. Process until very creamy.

Coconut/Macadamia Nut Crusted Salmon

This is a wonderfully sweet Hawaiian rendition of salmon I use for special occasions. It always gets rave reviews at The pH Miracle retreats! Serves 6.

Combine coconut, macadamias, salt and seasoning in food processor. Pulse chop to mix, then let the machine run until the mixture is finely ground and crumbly. Combine lime juice and coconut milk. Dip filets in the liquid, then into the coconut mixture to coat heavily. Press and pat the coating into the fish. In an electric frying pan on medium heat, fry 4–6 minutes, or until golden browned. Flip just once and fry on the other side until golden. If the fish is not done in the center, place the lid over the frying pan and steam until done. Lift each filet onto a serving platter with a spatula, taking care lest the coating crumbles off. Serve immediately.

6 salmon filets, thinly sliced (1/2 inch)

3 cups dehydrated unsweetened coconut flakes

3 cups raw macadamia nuts

1 teaspoon Real Salt

2 teaspoons Garlic Herb Bread Seasoning (Spice Hunter)

1 can coconut milk (Thai brand)

juice of three limes

grapeseed oil for frying

Wild Fajita Verde

By Lory Fabbi. Serve with Ensalada Mexico (p. 80). Serves 2–3.

Sauté peppers in a small non-stick pan wiped sparingly with oil; or grill on a Foreman type grill, 3–4 minutes until tender but still crunchy. Cook onion slices the same way until translucent. Warm tortilla in pan, remove and fill with peppers and onions. Top with cilantro, lime juice, avocado, rice or Kashi, and salsa verde.

1/2 red bell pepper, sliced in 1/4" wide long strips

1/2 green bell pepper, sliced in 1/4" wide long strips

1/2 small white or yellow onion, thinly sliced

1/2 cup cooked kashi pilaf (whole grains) or brown rice

2 tablespoons roasted green chilies diced

15 fresh cilantro leaves, rolled between fingers to crush

1/2 avocado sliced

salsa verde (I use Herdez brand—no vinegar)

dash of Bragg Liquid Aminos, if desired

2–3 sprouted wheat tortillas or fresh homemade spelt tortillas OR use large lettuce leaf in place of tortillas

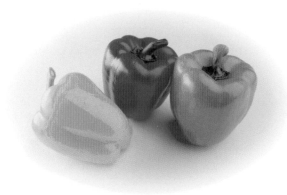

Tomato Asparagus Ratatouille

By Debra Jenkins. 1st place in transitional recipes, in the pH Miracle Recipe Contest. Serve on its own, or over wild rice, buckwheat, or spelt noodles. Makes a great alkaline anytime meal . . . even breakfast! Serves 2–4.

1 medium eggplant, peeled and cubed

1 cup asparagus, chopped

1/2 cup green beans, chopped

1 onion, chopped

1 clove garlic, minced or grated

1 small zucchini, sliced

3-4 fresh tomatoes

1-2 cups fresh spinach (optional)

1/4 cup olive oil (can use garlic flavored or rosemary for extra flavor)

1/4 teaspoon cayenne pepper

1/2 teaspoon garlic powder

1 teaspoon onion powder

1-2 teaspoons Mesquite Seasoning (Spice Hunter)

Real Salt and/or Bragg Liquid Aminos, to taste

Lightly sauté all vegetables except spinach in water in a skillet for 2-4 minutes. Stir in seasonings. Add spinach (if using) and stir for 30 seconds more. Remove from heat, pour olive oil over all, and spray with Bragg Liquid Aminos. Serve immediately.

Variation: Add a few white beans or tofu.

pH Pizza Delight

By David Martini. So fast, tasty and alkaline, you can enjoy this anytime. Serves 1–2.

1 sprouted wheat tortilla (large burrito size)

hummus

bell peppers in assorted colors

fresh cucumbers

fresh spinach

tofu

sun dried tomatoes packed in olive oil

Spice Hunter seasoning of your choice

Spread the hummus evenly on the tortilla. Cut the toppings into slices. (Roll spinach leaves up.) Place veggies on the hummus in whatever design or pattern you like. Sprinkle with your favorite Spice Hunter seasoning. Slice into wedges and enjoy!

Tomato Asparagus Ratatouille

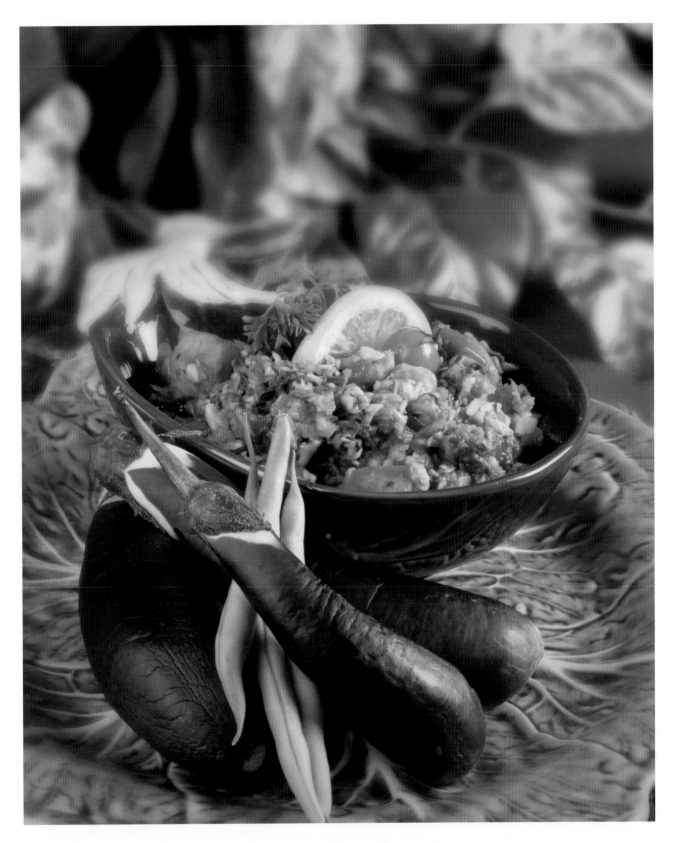

Fiesta Tacos El Alkalarian

By Kelly Anclien. Best Transitional recipe in pH Miracle recipe contest. Serves 4–6.

2 sprouted wheat tortillas

olive oil

Garlic Pepper (Spice Hunter)

fajita Seasoning

Real Salt

2 large tomatoes, peeled and seeded

5 tablespoons diced purple or red onion

2 sun dried tomatoes

1 1/2 teaspoons jalapeno pepper, seeded (mild salsa)

3 teaspoons fresh cilantro

2 garlic cloves minced

1 teaspoon fresh lemon juice

1/2 teaspoon ground pepper

2 avocados, mashed with a fork

1/2 teaspoon Mesquite Seasoning (Spice Hunter)

1/2 teaspoon Fajita Seasoning (Spice Hunter)

1/4 teaspoon Real Salt

1 16 oz. can refried beans

1–2 red bell peppers, sliced into strips

mixed greens to fill a salad bowl (about 1 medium bag, 16–24 oz.)

Line bottom oven rack with tin foil. Preheat oven to 350 degrees. Rub olive oil onto both sides of tortilla, and sprinkle one side with garlic pepper, fajita seasoning and salt. Hang each tortilla over 2 bars of the upper oven rack, to form the shape of tacos. (Any dripping oil will land on the tin foil.) Bake for 13 minutes, or until crisp. Meanwhile, make the salsa by blending tomatoes, onion, jalapeno, cilantro, garlic, lemon juice, and ground pepper in food processor to desired consistency. Use sun dried tomatoes if you like a sweeter, thicker salsa. Add Real Salt to taste. Make guacamole by stirring together avocado with mesquite and fajita seasoning and real salt. Assemble tacos with layers of refried beans, salsa, guacamole, red peppers and mixed greens.

Ensalada Mexico

By Lory Fabbi. The perfect compliment to Wild Fajita Verde. Or, to make it a main course on its own, serve with homemade tortilla chips and a dip made of refried beans, salsa, lime juice, and chopped onion, thinned slightly with water. Serves 2–3.

1/2 sliced red onion

1 chopped bell pepper

1/2 cup chopped jicama

2–3 radishes, sliced

1 ripe tomato, chopped

1/2 avocado, chopped

1/2 cup black or kidney beans (optional)

fresh salsa

Mix all but the last ingredient together, and top with your favorite fresh salsa (no vinegar).

Variation: Mix 1–2 tablespoons Vegannaise with 1/2 cup salsa in food processor or blender for a creamier dressing. Or, to boost the spiciness, add 1/4 of a jalepeno, peeled, seeded and chopped. (Warning: Wash hands immediately after handling jalapeno to remove hot pepper oil, which can otherwise really sting.)

Fiesta Tacos El Alkalarian

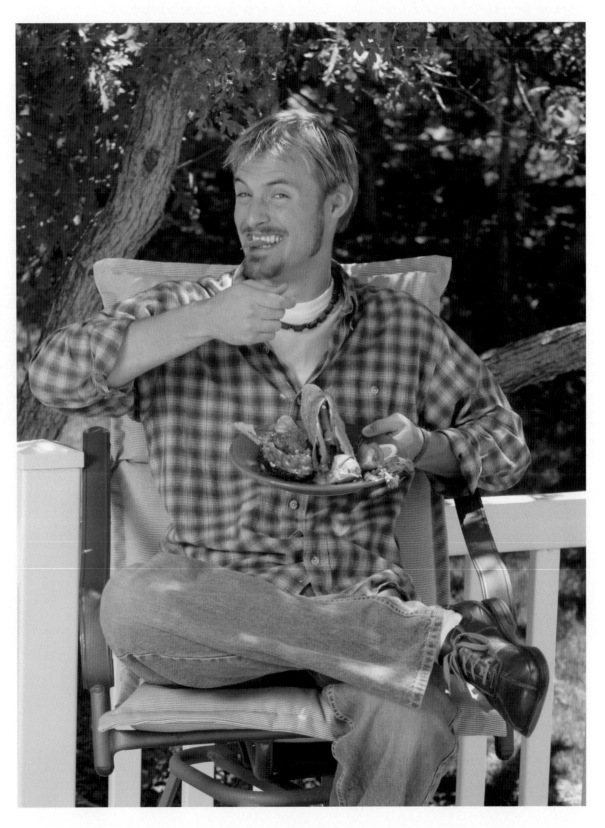

China Moon Vegetable Pasta with Coconut Lotus Sauce

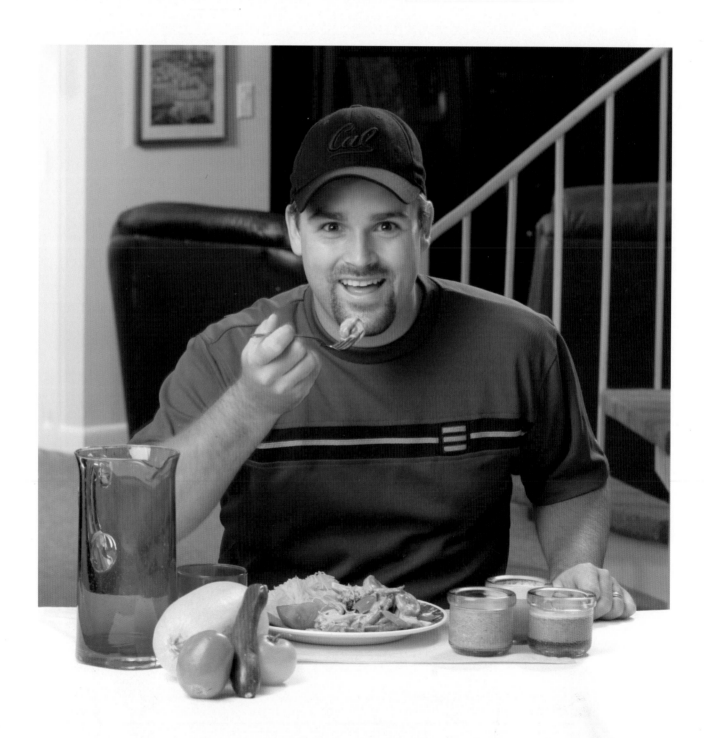

China Moon Vegetable Pasta with Coconut Lotus Sauce

By Lisa El-Kerdi. BEST IN SHOW recipe in The pH Miracle Recipe Contest. This colorful and flavorful dish is highly adaptable. Feel free to add vegetables of choice, modify according to season, and adjust quantities to suit the number of friends you are serving. Serves 6–8.

Cover lower oven rack with aluminum foil to catch any drippings. Preheat oven to 375–400 degrees. Make a one inch slit in top of spaghetti squash. Bake on upper oven rack for 30–50 minutes, or until squash gives to gentle pressure but is not mushy. Bring water to a boil in bottom of large pot with steamer tray, then reduce to simmer. Place vegetables in steamer starting with scallions and carrots and continuing in order listed above. Cover and steam gently for 3–5 minutes, then turn off heat. The stored heat will continue to cook the vegetables. Be careful not to let them get overdone! Cut squash in half and scoop seeds out of center. Run fork lengthwise along the inside of the squash to form "spaghetti", and scoop gently onto plates or into shallow bowls. When veggies are done, remove steamer tray from pot. (Save broth for a soup base!) Return vegetables to pot and toss gently with desired amount of sauce, and spoon on top of squash. Garnish with coconut and sesame seeds.

1 large or 2 small spaghetti squash

1 bunch scallions, cut in 2" diagonals

1 carrot, thinly sliced

1–2 cups broccoli florets

1/2 lb. asparagus, cut in 2" diagonals

1 red bell pepper, sliced

2 yellow squash, sliced

1 zucchini, sliced

4–6 tiny bok choy, leaves separated, or 1/2 stalk large bok choy, sliced

1/2 lb. snow peas

1–1 1/2 cups coconut lotus sauce (recipe follows)

shredded unsweetened coconut

black sesame seeds

Coconut Lotus Sauce

Besides making China Moon vegetable pasta, you can use this versatile sauce on a stir fry or as a dressing or dip.

Blend first three ingredients in food processor or VitaMix. Add Bragg Liquid Aminos and blend until smooth. Pour into jar, then add oils, coconut milk, water and shake. Thin with water, carrot juice or vegetable broth if desired. Store in refrigerator.

Variations:
* For Thai lotus sauce, add juice of one lime, 2 tablespoons fresh or 1 teaspoon dried lemongrass, 1 teaspoon fresh or 1/2 teaspoon dried basil and chopped fresh cilantro if desired.
* For basic lotus sauce, omit coconut milk and increase flaxseed oil to 1/4–1/3 cup.
* For lotus dressing, add to 1/2 cup basic lotus sauce 1/4 cup lime juice, 1 1/2 cups flaxseed or untoasted sesame oil, 1/2 carrot (optional) and 1/2 sweet onion (optional), and blend until smooth.
* For Indonesian dipping sauce, add to 3/4 cup basic lotus sauce 1 cup almond butter, 1/4 teaspoon crushed red pepper (or to taste), and 1/2–1 cup unsweetened coconut milk to reach desired consistency.

2" piece of ginger root, peeled and sliced

2 large cloves garlic

1/2 teaspoon crushed red pepper flakes (adjust to desired heat)

1/2 cup Bragg Liquid Aminos (or more to taste)

2 tablespoons toasted sesame oil

2 tablespoons flaxseed oil

1/4 cup water, carrot juice, or vegetable broth (optional)

Real Salt, to taste

1 c. unsweetened coconut milk (I prefer Thai Kitchen), or more if desired

North African Bean Stew

By Lisa El-Kerdi. Best in Show in the pH Miracle Recipe Contest. This rich and exotic stew is sure to spice up any gathering. Serve with Moroccan Mint Salad (p. 44). Serves 4–6.

1 1/2 cups uncooked 7 bean and barley mix (or any mix of dried beans), soaked overnight, rinsed, and drained

1 bay leaf

1/8 teaspoon cinnamon

4 cloves garlic

2 onions, quartered

4 carrots, cut into chunks

4 stalks celery, cut into chunks

1 large or 2 small eggplant

Real Salt

1 red bell pepper

1 yellow bell pepper

1/2 teaspoon turmeric

1 teaspoon coriander

1 teaspoon cumin

1/2 teaspoon cardamom

1/8 teaspoon black pepper

1/8 teaspoon cayenne

3–4 cloves garlic, pressed

2 or 3 yellow squash

2 or 3 zucchini

4 chopped tomatoes or 1 box Pomi chopped tomatoes

1 teaspoon Real Salt

olive oil

Cover beans with 2 1/2" water in large pot and add bay leaf and cinnamon. Bring to boil and skim off foam. Reduce to low heat and simmer, covered, for 30 minutes. Chop garlic, onions, carrots, and celery in food processor. Add to beans after 30 minutes cooking. Simmer until beans are cooked, 1–1 1/2 hour. Cube and generously salt eggplant. Let sit 1/2–1 hour. Chop peppers. Rinse eggplant and squeeze out juices. While eggplant is salting, sauté spices in olive oil. Add to beans. Add eggplant and peppers. Simmer 1/2 hour. Cut squashes in half lengthwise and slice. Add to stew. Simmer 10 minutes. Add tomatoes and salt to stew. Simmer 10 minutes. Adjust salt to taste. Ladle into deep bowls and top each serving with 1 tablespoon olive oil (or to taste).

Can't Get Enough Eggplant

Recipe By Myra Marvez. Serves 1–2.

1 eggplant

olive oil

Celtic salt

1 finely chopped onion, size chosen according to taste and size of eggplant(s)

Roast eggplant on open fire till it is mostly cooked. Cool and peel all burned skin off. Chop eggplant into small pieces. Finely mince the onion. Place eggplant in bowl, add onion, olive oil, salt, and mix well.

Super Stuffed Tomatoes

By Frances Fujii. This makes a beautiful presentation. Serves 2–4.

Soak black beans overnight. Put in medium sized pot, add 2" water and bring to a boil. Simmer for 1 hour or until tender. (Can use beans whole or slightly mashed.) Season with seasoning salt and set aside. Cook wild/brown rice, set aside. Lightly sauté onions and garlic and macadamia oil. Add greens and small amount of water and steam-fry until just tender, about 5 minutes. Season with Bragg Liquid Aminos and set aside. Lightly sauté tofu in same pan and add seasoning salt to taste. Scoop out tomatoes. Dice scooped out sections and set aside. Bake hollowed-out tomatoes at 300 degrees for 5–10 minutes to warm. (Do not over-bake or the tomatoes will get too soft). On individual serving plates, create a bottom "ring" of wild rice, with a second ring of seasoned black beans on top of it. Place a hollowed tomato in the center of the double-decker ring. Sprinkle tofu cubes around on top of the beans/rice at the base of the tomato and stuff the tomato with greens (spill greens to over-flow the top of the tomato if desired). Sprinkle the raw diced tomatoes on top of the greens, drizzle a little Udo's or olive oil and serve. Note: If you like garlic, you can mix in roasted garlic to the warm cooked brown rice before serving.

6 medium-sized tomatoes

1 cup (dry) black beans

2 pkg. firm tofu

2 lb. Swiss chard, coarsely chopped (may substitute kale, spinach, beet greens or other preferred leafy green vegetable)

2 cups (uncooked) wild rice (or use 1/2 brown and 1/2 wild rice)

4 cloves garlic diced

1 medium onion diced

Bragg Liquid Aminos

vegetable seasoning salt (I like Herbamare)

macadamia oil

Udo's oil or olive oil

Robio's Burrito

By Robio. This burrito would make a great meal anytime . . . even for breakfast. You can add or subtract and cut/slice/dice the items listed below to your own specifications. This recipe is so versatile, and you can add your own spin on it every time to make it delicious and entertaining. Serves 1.

Place the refried beans directly down the middle of the tortilla, then add the other toppings as you like. Fold like a taco or roll up like a burrito.

1 sprouted wheat , spelt, or grain tortilla

organic refried beans

1 avocado

Herdez salsa (hot, medium, or mild)

lettuce

tomato

green pepper

jalapenos

onions

California white basmati rice seasoned with Spanish spices (optional)

Coconut Curry Salmon Chowder

This is a sweet rich dish. Serves 4.

1 lb. fresh salmon

1 teaspoon Real Salt

1–2 teaspoons Garlic Herb Bread Seasoning
(Spice Hunter)

1 yellow onion

8 stalks celery

6 carrots

2 cans coconut milk (I use Thai brand)

1/2 teaspoon Thai green curry paste (I use
Thai brand)

1–2 pkg. powdered stevia (I use the stevia
with fiber) (Note: If using straight stevia,
then use much less)

1 cup fresh coconut

1/2 teaspoon vanilla (I use Frontier brand
with no alcohol)

1 cup fresh peas from the pod (optional)

1 cup fresh spinach (optional)

Sprinkle fish with some Real Salt and Garlic Herb Bread Seasoning and steam fry. Or, if you prefer, use some grapeseed oil and fry until cooked through but still moist. Cut into small bite-size pieces and set aside. Cut the onion, carrots, and celery into bite-size chunks, and put into a soup pot and steam until bright and chewy. (Do not overcook). Add the coconut milk, green curry paste, vanilla, and stevia and stir into mix. Add salmon. Take 1/3 of the whole ingredients and puree in blender and then return to the soup for a thick colorful base. Add fresh peas from the pod and/or fresh spinach towards the end if you like, and warm before serving.

Energizer-Alkalizer Breakfast

By Susan Lee Traft. This breakfast keeps you going strong and feeling awesome for several hours. Serves 2.

1/4 cup chopped red pepper

1/4 cup chopped onion

1 clove of minced garlic

2 cups of mixed veggies (such as Swiss
chard, broccoli, green beans, pea pods,
zucchini, slices of carrot, etc.)

1 to 3 tablespoons of golden flaxseeds
(ground in coffee grinder, tastes like
bread crumbs)

1 tablespoon Udo's oil

Bragg Liquid Aminos, to taste

Bring water to a simmer under steamer basket in pot. Add red pepper, onion, garlic and mixed veggies all at once into steamer basket and cover. Lightly steam (no more than 5 minutes). Immediately remove veggies from heat and put into salad bowl. Add oil, ground flaxseed and the Bragg Liquid Aminos. Mix well.

Coconut Curry Salmon Chowder

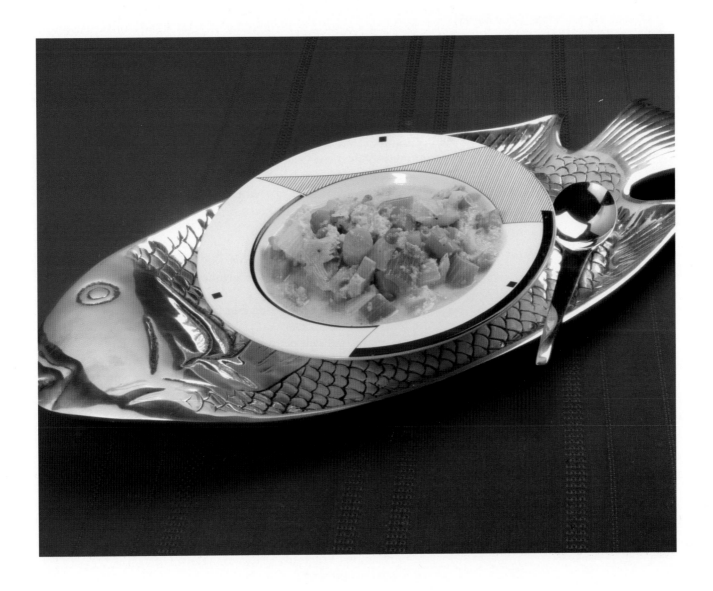

Veggie Tofu Loaf

This is a wonderfully colorful and nutritious way to enjoy tofu at any meal or even snack time. It's great steaming hot from the oven or sliced cold or broken up over a salad. Use the firmest tofu type for best holding results. I use Nigari brand Extra Firm. For a binder, I use Mauk Family Farms Wheat Free Crusts, a blend of gold and brown flax seeds, sesame seeds and sunflower seeds, with garlic, onion, celery seed, red bell pepper, parsley, sea salt and pepper, dehydrated at 105 degrees, and process them in my food processor until they are a powder consistency. The flax, sunflower, and sesame seeds add extra flavor and healthy fats. This is also a favorite dish served at the pH Miracle Retreats. Serves 6.

1 lb. firm or extra firm tofu

1/2 to 1 teaspoon Real Salt (or to taste)

5 teaspoons Mexican Seasonings (Spice Hunter)

2 teaspoons Vegetable Rub (Spice Hunter)

4 teaspoon sun dried tomatoes, minced (Melissa Brand packed in olive oil)

1/2 red bell pepper diced

2 tablespoons diced celery

2 tablespoons diced soaked almonds

2 tablespoons raw wheat-free crusts, ground to powder (Mauk Family Farms)

Use the food processor to dice all ingredients that need dicing. Then place all ingredients in food processor and pulse chop until well mixed. Place on a grapeseed oiled pan and mold into a loaf or two smaller loafs, about 2 inches in height. Brush some grapeseed oil over the top of the loaf and sprinkle The Zip over the top. Bake at 400 degrees for 20–30 minutes or until lightly browned on top. Serve warm or let it chill over night. Slice and serve cold. Serves 6.

Variation 1: Garlic Veggie Tofu Loaf.
1 lb. extra firm Nigari tofu
1/2 to 1 teaspoon Real Salt
2–4 roasted cloves of garlic
2 tablespoons Spice House Dehydrated Veggie Granules
4 teaspoons diced celery
4 teaspoons diced red bell pepper
2 tablespoons ground raw wheat-free crusts
Top the loaf with Garlic Herb Bread Seasoning.

Variation 2: Buckwheat Veggie Tofu Loaf
The binder for this variation is raw buckwheat flour. Grind raw buckwheat in your blender or grinder to make this flour fresh.
1 lb. extra firm tofu
6 teaspoons Vegetable Seasoning (Spice Hunter)
6 teaspoons diced celery
3 teaspoons red bell pepper
3 teaspoons diced sun dried tomato
5 teaspoons Garlic Herb Bread Seasoning (Spice Hunter)
1/2–1 teaspoon Real Salt
3 teaspoons raw buckwheat, ground to flour
Top the loaf with 2 teaspoons ground raw wheat free crusts (reference above).

Variation 3: Basil Veggie Tofu Loaf
1 lb. extra firm Nigari tofu
1/2–1 teaspoon Real Salt
4 teaspoons diced celery
4 teaspoons diced red bell pepper
2 tablespoons Vegetable Seasoning (Spice Hunter)
4 teaspoons ground flax seeds
4 teaspoons ground soaked almonds
6–8 teaspoons fresh diced basil
Top the loaf with Garlic Herb Bread Seasoning.

Variation 4: Quinoa Veggie Tofu Loaf
1 lb. extra firm Nigari tofu
1 tablespoon Pesto Seasoning (Spice Hunter)
2 tablespoons diced celery
2 tablespoons diced red bell pepper
4 teaspoons minced sun dried tomato (packed in olive oil)
1 heaping tablespoon of quinoa ground flour (grind in your blender)
Top the loaf with dehydrated veggie granules (Spice House).

Veggie Tofu Loaf

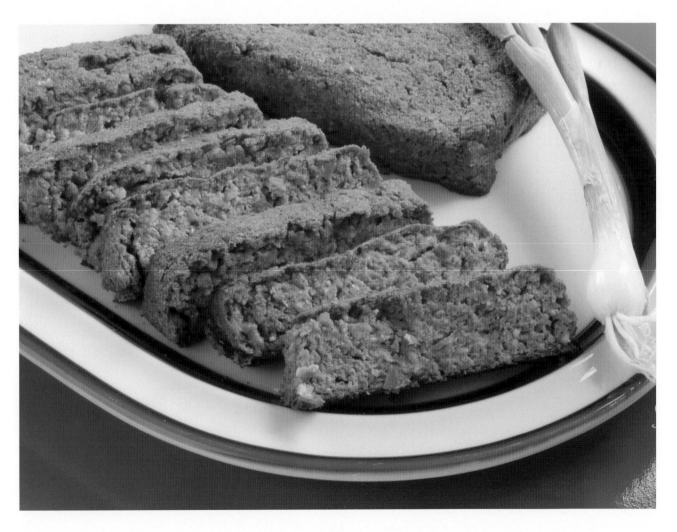

Steamed Fish and Greens in Coconut Water

Serves 4.

Place the fish, skin side down, in a non-stick frying pan and steam fry with the lid on until the fish is cooked through but also moist. Half-way through, take the lid off and sprinkle the fish with Real Salt and Garlic Herb Bread Seasoning (Spice Hunter). When the fish is done, take out on a plate and set aside. Take the skin off the fish and discard but leave any oils from the fish in the pan. Place the thinly sliced ginger in the oiled pan and cook until the ginger is browned. Add all other ingredients except cilantro and steam in the pan with the lid on until bright green and softened. Add the fish and the cilantro back in and steam one or two more minutes before serving.

1 lb. fresh salmon, trout, or red snapper filet with skin on

1 tablespoon fresh ginger, cut in thin slices or grated

1 cup yellow chives

1/2 cup green chives

1/2 cup cilantro

4 cups fresh kale

2 tablespoons Bragg Liquid Aminos

1/2–1 cup fresh coconut water (sweet) taken from a young fresh coconut*

Real Salt to taste

* (To get coconut water, I use a clean screwdriver and a hammer to make two holes into the top of a coconut. Pour the water out into a measuring cup. Then break open the coconut with the hammer and a sharp meat cleaver to get to the fresh coconut meat.)

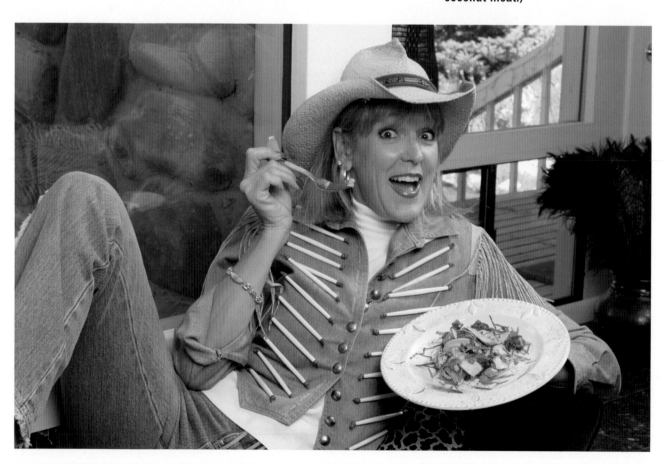

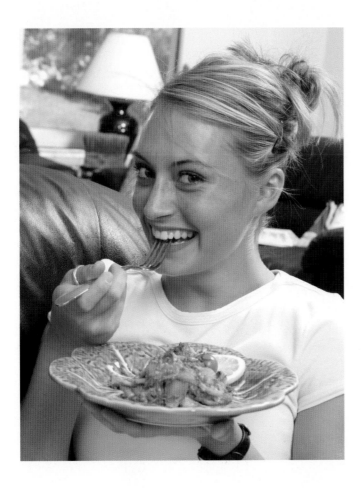

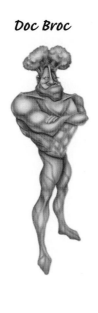

Doc Broc

Doc Broc Stalks—Coyote Style

The good news is that when Dr. Young first tried this dish, he thought he was eating fried potatoes! I love it when I can fake him out! The even better news is that this tasty treat is actually made of broccoli. Even my 15 year old Alex (our perpetual transitional boy) always asks for seconds and thirds of these.

Place sliced onion and sliced broccoli stalks pieces in a non stick fry pan together and steam fry for few minutes until onions and broccoli heat up and steam so they slip and slide around the pan. Add the grapeseed oil and stir veggies on high heat while they brown and become somewhat roasted. Once they are evenly fry roasted, turn down the heat to low and add 1/2 cup of the creamy tomato soup (more or less depending on how much sauce you want in with your stalks, you can always add the other 1/2 later). Then sprinkle in seasonings to coat the stalks and onions. Stir well to distribute all the seasonings evenly. Last sprinkle in the amount of desired soy parmesan and stir once more to mix well.

- 6 long broccoli stalks peeled and thinly sliced, about 1/8 of an inch
- 1 yellow onion thinly sliced and chopped
- 2 tablespoon grapeseed oil
- 1/2 to 1 cup creamy tomato soup (see recipe on p. 51)
- 1–2 teaspoons Garlic Herb Bread Seasoning (Spice Hunter)
- 1–2 teaspoons Seafood Grill and Broil Seasoning (Spice Hunter)
- 1–2 teaspoons Mesquite Seasoning (Spice Hunter)
- 1/2 teaspoon ground yellow mustard
- 1–3 teaspoons soy parmesan (alternative) cheese, dairy free (I use Soymage Vegan Parmesan)

Doc Broc Brunch

This is a hearty Deep Green dish that has plenty of crunch with the broccoli stalks and soaked almonds added. Perfect for a brunch or side dish. Serves 6.

1 yellow onion

2 cloves fresh garlic

3 large heads of broccoli

1 lb. of young green string beans

1 small bowl of soaked almonds

grapeseed or olive oil

Real Salt to taste

Trim and peel broccoli stalks. Then cut broccoli into bite size pieces. Trim and break green beans into bite size pieces. Lightly steam broccoli and green beans until bright green. In a food processor, pulse chop the onion and garlic until fine, then set aside. Put soaked almonds into the food processor with an S blade and pulse chop into almond slivers. In an electric fry pan, place oil and add onion/garlic mixture and sauté for a few minutes. Add steamed broccoli/green beans and stir fry to mix in with the onions and garlic. Add slivered soaked almonds and continue to mix well. Put lid on electric fry pan and continue to steam for a few minutes longer if softer veggies are desired. Add Real Salt to taste.

Doc Broc

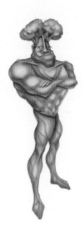

Doc Broc Casserole

Serves 4–6.

1 pkg. Smart Ground by LiteLife (soy protein substitute)

florets from 2 large bunches of broccoli (save leaves and stocks out, peel and clean stocks)

1 small bunch of fresh basil or tarragon stemmed and minced

1 cup soft tofu

1 teaspoon ground mustard seed

2/3 cup olive oil

1–2 cups roasted or soaked and re-dehydrated almonds for topping

Real Salt and The Zip, to taste

Steam broccoli with a little water in a covered pan for about 4–5 minutes until broccoli is bright green and just crisp/tender. In a food processor, process the broccoli leaves and stocks until very fine (scrape down sides if necessary). Then add the soft tofu, mustard and basil into the food processor with the fine broccoli mixture and process. With the processor running, slowly add the olive oil until mixture is well emulsified and creamy. In a large electric fry pan, heat a small amount of oil and add the soy Smart Ground, crumble it up and fry it for a couple of minutes, then add the steamed broccoli and pour the creamy sauce from the processor over the top and stir in well. Use roasted slivered or dehydrated almonds and cut them up into small bits in the food processor for extra crunch . . . Then sprinkle over the top of the broccoli mixture and serve. Or return the lid to the fry pan and steam the mixture a bit to soften the almonds and broccoli more. Add Real Salt and The Zip to taste.

Transitional variaton: Take one bag of Garlic Onion Olive Oil potato chips by Terra brand and mash them with a rolling pin. Sprinkle them over the top instead of the almonds. Put lid on and steam a bit to soften the chips.   Kids love this one!

Doc Broc Casserole

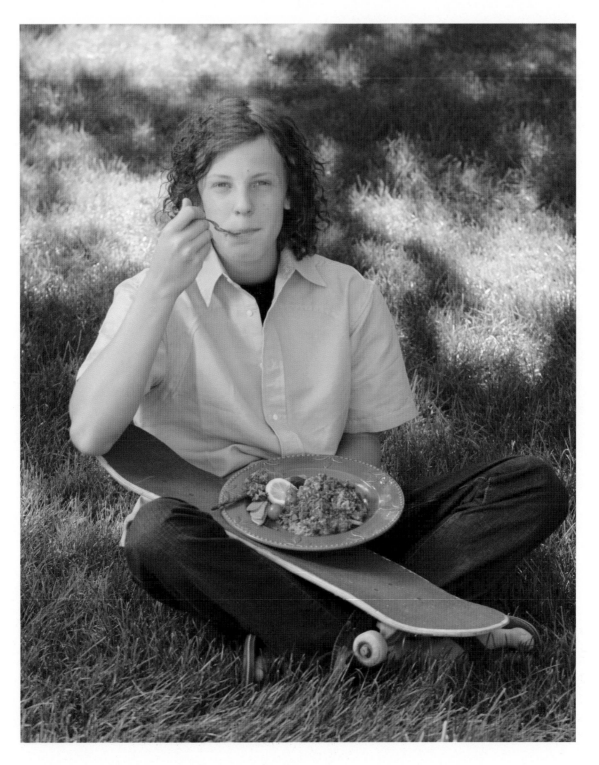

"Train up a child in the way he should go: and when he is old, he will not depart from it."

Proverbs 22:6

Roasted Veggie Pizzas

I developed this recipe from "Shelley's Super Wraps" (from The pH Miracle*), roasting the veggies, and crisping the tortillas. These are by far the favorite dinner at pH Miracle retreats. Feel free to add to or change the veggies you use in any way that appeals to you. Eggplant, bok choy, celery, and snow peas, anyone? Serves 8–10.*

3 red bell peppers

2–3 orange bell peppers

1–2 green bell peppers

2 sweet onions (I use yellow)

20–30 whole pieces (cloves) of garlic

4 yellow crook neck squash

3 zucchinis

2 large heads of broccoli, cut into flowerets

1–2 heads of cauliflower, chopped

3 avocados, sliced

1 package (6–8) sprouted wheat tortillas

2 cups hummus (or 1 recipe of Yummus Hummus from *The pH Miracle*)

2 cups non-dairy pesto (or 1 recipe of Spring's Pesto from *The PH Miracle*)

1 8–12 oz. tube sun-dried tomato paste (or make your own by whirling 12–15 sun-dried tomatoes in a food processor)

1 lb. bag pine nuts or slivered almonds (optional)

Preheat broiler. Cut the veggies, except avocado, into bite sized chunks. Place on cookie sheets and lightly sprinkle with grapeseed oil. Broil until lightly browned on the edges, about 15 minutes. Meanwhile, spread a thick layer of hummus and pesto on each tortilla. Top with generous amounts of roasted veggies, and top with avocado and some squirts of sun-dried tomato paste. Sprinkle with nuts if desired. Place under broiler until tortillas have crisped and veggies are sizzling hot, and serve immediately.

CHAPTER 3

Roof

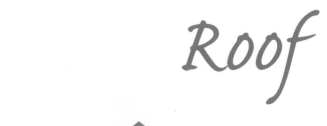

The best blood transfusion you can get is from the blood of green grasses and plants.
Dr. Robert O. Young

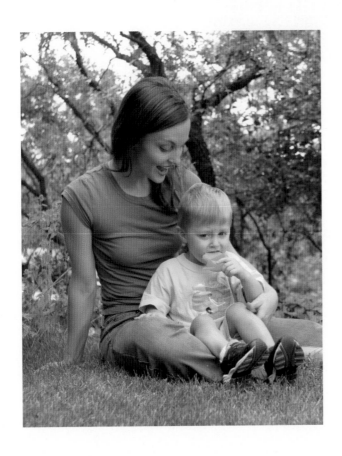

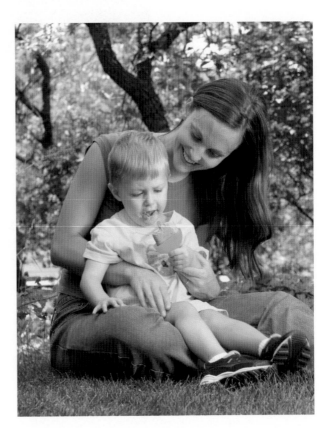

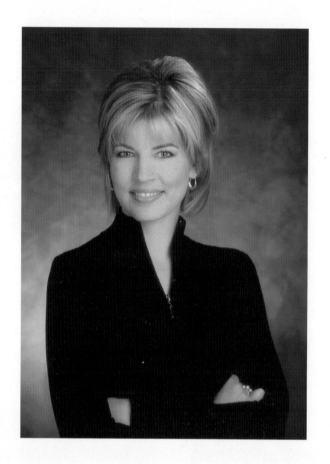

"It is clear to me how this way of eating
can totally change your life.
It's a revelation, a way of looking at the world in a
new light. It affects the way we look at ourselves,
and disease, and how the food we put into our
bodies affects everything we do."

**Jane Clayson
CBS News**

Almond Chili Sauce

By Roxy Boelz. 3rd place, pH Miracle Recipe Contest. Serves 2–4.

Blend all ingredients together in blender till smooth. Add the water gradually, until you get the consistency you desire.

- 1/2 cup raw almond butter
- 1 tablespoon fresh ginger, grated
- 2 tablespoons lemon juice
- 1 clove of garlic
- 1 tablespoon Bragg Liquid Aminos
- 1 chili, such as Serrano
- 1/4 cup water

Mock Sour Cream

By Roxy Boelz. 3rd place, pH Miracle Recipe Contest. Serves 2–4.

Blend all ingredients until smooth. Add water gradually to get the consistency you want.

- 3/4 cup coconut meat
- 1/3 cup Brazil nuts (soaked overnight)
- 3 tablespoons olive oil
- 2 tablespoons lemon juice
- 1 tablespoon water
- 1/2 teaspoon Real Salt

Sunny Spread

By Roxy Boelz. 3rd place, the pH Miracle Recipe Contest. Serves 2–4.

1 cup sunflower seeds (soaked for 6 hours or overnight)

1 cup almonds (soaked for 6 hours or overnight)

2 tablespoons lemon juice

1/2 cup fresh herbs of choice (parsley, basil, cilantro, etc.)

1 tablespoon dulse flakes

Process sunflower seeds and almonds in food processor. Add remaining ingredients except dulse flakes and stir well. Sprinkle on the dulse flakes.

Variations: For garlic flavor, add chopped garlic to lemon juice and herbs, then combine with sunflower/almond mixture. Use 1 teaspoon kelp instead of dulse flakes, adding kelp in the food processor with the rest of the ingredients.

Tofu Hummus

By Debra Jenkins. 1st place, Transitional Recipes, in the pH Miracle Recipe Contest. Serves 2–3.

8 oz. tofu

1/2 cup raw tahini

1/2 lemon, juiced

1 teaspoon cumin

2–3 sun dried peppers or tomatoes

1 clove garlic

1/2 teaspoon Real Salt

Blend all ingredients together.

Almond Gravy

By Debra Jenkins. 1st place, Transitional Recipes, the pH Miracle Recipe Contest.
This is good over buckwheat, rice, veggie burgers, vegetables, salmon and more. Serves 2–3.

Blend ingredients together. Then warm over high heat, stirring constantly until thickened, about 3 minutes.

2 cups water
1/2 cup almonds (soaked and blanched, if preferred)
2 tablespoons arrowroot powder
2 teaspoons onion powder
2 tablespoons grapeseed oil
1/2 teaspoon Real Salt

Tofu "Whipped Cream"

By Debra Jenkins. 1st place, Transitional Recipes, in the pH Miracle Recipe Contest.
Use this as a topping in place of whipped cream, over warmed grains or dessert selections from this chapter like the key lime or pumpkin pie, also by Debra. Serves 2–4.

Drain tofu thoroughly. Combine tofu, vanilla, stevia and lemon juice in food processor and blend. Add water or almond milk as needed to create a smooth consistency (should take only a few tablespoons). To make whipped cream stiffer, add psyllium or agar. Refrigerate until chilled.

Variation: Flavor with cinnamon.

1/2 pound (8 oz.) Silken Tofu
2 teaspoon Frontier non-alcoholic vanilla
1/8 teaspoon stevia
1 tablespoon lemon juice
water or almond milk
1 1/2 teaspoon psyllium or agar flakes (optional)

Nutty Cream Topping

By Debra Jenkins. 1st place winner of Best Transitional Recipes, in the pH Miracle Recipe Contest. Serves 1–2.

1/2 cup almonds
1/3 cup boiling water
1/2 teaspoon lemon juice
stevia

In a blender or coffee grinder, grind almonds to a fine powder. Add water, juice and stevia to taste (about 2–3 drops of liquid or one packet). Blend on high till smooth and creamy. Chill for an hour or two.

Variation: Flavor with cinnamon, almond or maple flavoring (be sure to get the flavors without alcohol).

Chips and Salsa

By Kelly Anclien. 1st place of BEST transitional recipes, in the pH Miracle Recipe Contest.
This recipe is great served as part of Kelly's other recipe, Fiesta Tacos El Alkalarian Sprouted wheat tortillas. Serves 4.

Chips:
sprouted wheat tortillas
olive oil
garlic pepper
fajita seasoning
Real Salt

Salsa:
2 large tomatoes
5 tablespoons diced purple or red onion
1 1/2 jalapeno peppers, seeded and chopped
    (mild salsa)
3 teaspoons chopped fresh cilantro
2 garlic cloves minced
1 teaspoon fresh lemon juice
Real Salt, to taste
1/2 teaspoon pepper
2 sun dried tomatoes (optional)

Preheat oven to 350 degrees. Rub oil onto both sides of each tortilla, and sprinkle one side with spices (those above, or any combination you dream up). Use a pizza cutter to slice each tortilla into 8 triangles. Bake on a cookie sheet for 13 minutes, or until crispy. Meanwhile, make the salsa. Place the remaining ingredients into a food processor and blend to desired consistency. Use the sun dried tomatoes if desired to sweeten and thicken the salsa.

Halva Coconut Freezer Balls

By Debra Jenkins. 1st place transitional recipes, in The pH Miracle Recipe Contest.

Melt coconut butter and mix all ingredients together. Drop teaspoons full onto a small cookie sheet or plate. Freeze for 15–20 minutes. Transfer to a freezer bag or container and eat as a luscious, quick dessert right from the freezer or fridge.

Variation: Use 3 tablespoons almond butter in place of tahini.

3 tablespoons raw tahini
1 tablespoon vanilla
1 tablespoon Garden of Life coconut butter (melted)
3 tablespoons fresh grated coconut
1/8 teaspoon stevia
2 tablespoons spelt flour

Coconut Macadamia Nut Cookies

By Debra Jenkins. 1st place transitional recipes, The pH Miracle Recipe Contest.

Mix dry ingredients together. Melt coconut butter and mix with water and vanilla. Pour liquid ingredients over dry ingredients and mix well. Drop onto cookie sheets and press very flat. Bake at 350 degrees for 15–20 minutes. Cool completely.

Egg substitute 1 (equivalent to about 1 egg)
1/3 cup water
1 tablespoon flaxseeds
Gently boil in a saucepan for about 5 minutes. Look for the consistency of a raw egg white. Do NOT use high heat or mixture will gel. You might want to strain this before using, depending on the recipe you are using. It is not necessary here.

Egg substitute 2 (equivalent to about 1 egg)
2/3 cup water
1–2 tablespoons agar flakes
Stir to combine.

Egg substitute 3 (equivalent to about 1 egg)
Use arrowroot flour in place of agar or flaxseeds in either recipe above.

1/2 cup fresh ground spelt flour (from spelt flakes—I use my old coffee grinder)
1/2 cup fresh grated coconut
1/4 cup chopped macadamia nuts
4 tablespoons Garden of Life coconut butter (melted)
egg substitute, equivalent to 2 eggs (see below – make a double recipe)
1/2 teaspoon Real Salt
1/4 teaspoon nutmeg
1/2 teaspoon cardamom
1 1/2 tablespoons non-alcoholic Frontier vanilla
1 teaspoon cinnamon
stevia, to taste (I use 2–3 packets or 1/4 teaspoon stevia powder)

Decadent Dill Spread

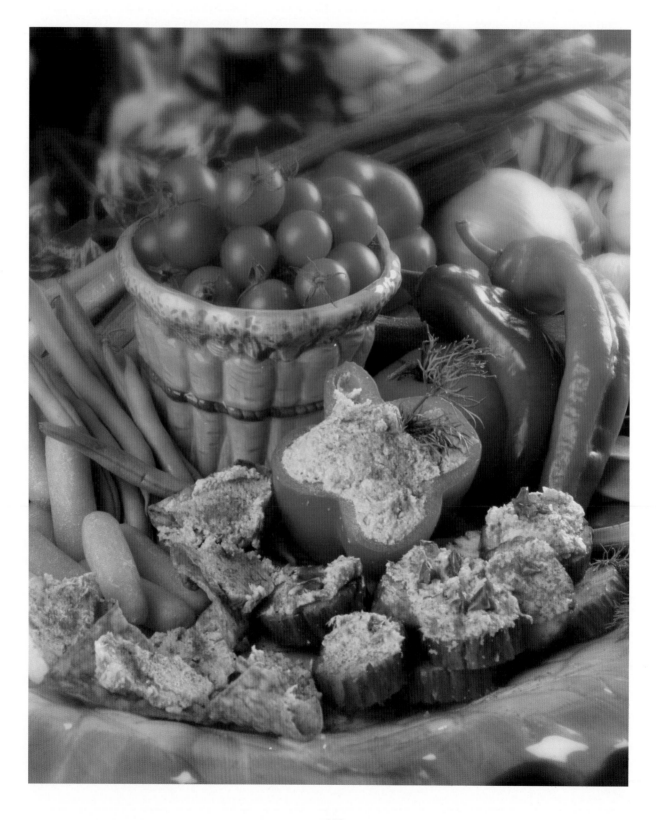

Decadent Dill Spread

By Eric Prouty. 2nd place for alkalizing recipes, in the pH Miracle Recipe Contest

Spread on cucumber slices, celery stalks, sushi nori paper (for veggie rolls), flax crackers, or sprouted tortillas (for veggie wraps). Serves 4.

Use Green Star/Green Life or Champion Juicer with plug attachment for nut butters. Add seeds, garlic and then onion. Mix with other ingredients in a bowl.

2 cups soaked sunflower seeds

3 cloves garlic

1/3 onion

2 tablespoons olive oil

1 tablespoon Bragg Liquid Aminos (or 1/2 to 1 teaspoon Real Salt)

1 teaspoon dill

Tomata Tostada Basilicious

By Dianne Ellsworth. Use your favorite pre-made tortillas for this recipe. Or, make your own. Dianne likes to tweak the Shelley's Super Tortillas recipe The pH Miracle by adding about 20 sun dried tomatoes, an additional 2–4 basil leaves, a peeled and seeded roasted green chili, and reducing the amount of coconut milk or water to achieve the correct consistency for dough.

In a food processor put oil, lime juice, garlic and tahini and process until smooth. Add beans, sun dried tomatoes and seasonings and process until creamy. You may need to thin with extra water (from beans) to desired consistency. Spread hummus on tortillas, add a layer of tomato slices and a layer of guacamole, and garnish with sliced basil leaves.

2–3 tablespoons olive oil

juice of 1 lime

1–2 garlic cloves, minced

1/8 – 1/4 cup raw tahini

1 17–oz. jar garbanzo beans, drained (save water)

20–22 sun dried tomatoes packed in olive oil

8–10 basil leaves (plus additional for garnish)

Real Salt, to taste

1/2–1 teaspoon Garlic Herb Bread Seasoning (Spice Hunter)

1/2–1 teaspoon cumin

Zip (Spice Hunter), to taste

2–6 tortillas

1–2 tomatoes, sliced

1–2 cups guacamole

Cherry Tomatoes AvoRado Style

This is a great appetizer or hors d'oeuvre, or it could be served as a salad course. Serves 2–4.

1 pint cherry tomatoes
juice from 1/2 lime
1 avocado
1/2 teaspoon dried onion
1 tablespoon minced cilantro
1/8 teaspoon Zip (Spice Hunter) (use more if you like extra spicy)
1/8 teaspoon Real Salt
dehydrated vegetable granules (make your own or buy them)

Slice off tomato tops and use a melon ball spoon to scoop out seeds and pulp of tomatoes. Drain on paper towels upside down. In food processor with an S blade add remaining ingredients and pulse chop into a well mixed chunky consistency. Fill tomato shells with mixture and sprinkle dehydrated veggie granules on top. Serve chilled.

Onion-Flax Crackers

By Roxy Boelz. 3rd place, The pH Miracle Recipe Contest. Serves 6–8.

2 cups sprouted sunflower seeds
1 cup chopped onion
1/2 cup fresh lemon juice or grapefruit juice (not sweet)
1 garlic clove
1/4 cup golden flaxseed
2 tablespoons raw almond butter or tahini
Real Salt, to taste
1/4 cup fennel seeds or sesame seeds or caraway seeds
1/2 cup filtered water

Purée all ingredients in food processor. Pour onto teflex sheets for dehydrator. Dehydrate at 105–110 degrees for 12 hours or to the desired crispness. Periodically score the batter as it dehydrates so you can separate more easily into crackers when done.

Onion-Flax Crackers

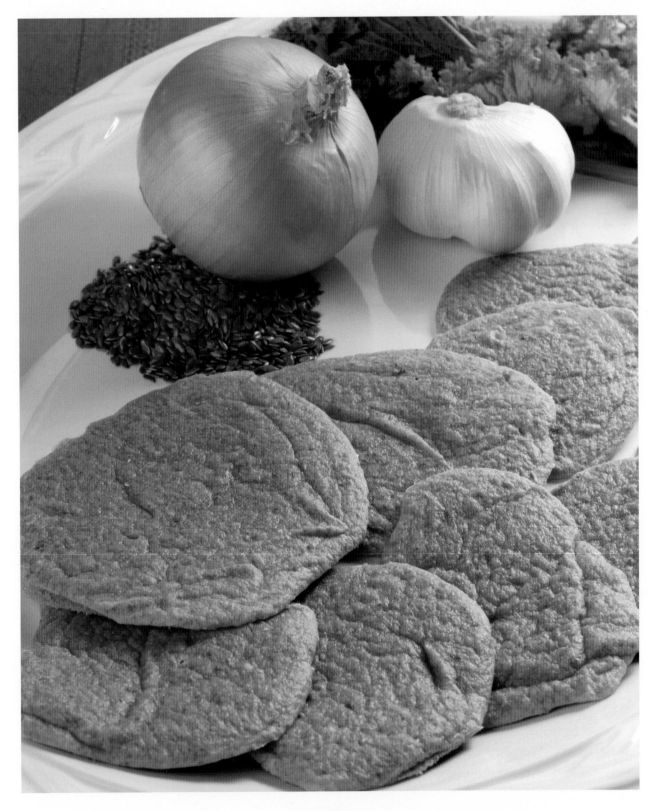

Red Pepper Dessert Boats

By Eric Prouty. 2nd place in Alkalarian recipes, in The pH Miracle Recipe Contest. Serves 4–6.

1–1/2 cups soaked sunflower seeds

1 tablespoon pumpkin seed oil

1 teaspoon cinnamon

7 drops liquid stevia mixed with 1 teaspoon water

2 red bell peppers

Use Green Star/Green Life or Champion Juicer with plug attachment for nut butters to process sunflower seeds. Mix in oil, cinnamon, and stevia and water. Slice red bell peppers in half vertically, core, and slice in slices (top to bottom, 1/2"–1" wide). Spread slices with sunflower seed mixture.

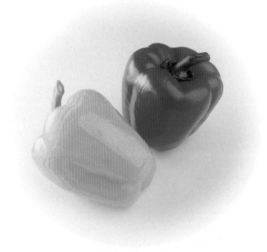

Red Pepper Jelly

By Cheri Freeman. 3rd place, Transitional recipes in the pH Miracle Recipe Contest. This keeps a few days in the fridge, or you can freeze it to use later. For a great snack, make little triangle sandwiches with warm sprouted wheat tortillas cut into quarters, almond butter and red pepper jelly. Yield: 1 1/2 cups; Serves 4.

2 red bell peppers

30 drops stevia (or to taste)

1/2 cup plus 3 tablespoons water

4 teaspoons Pomona's Universal Pectin

4 teaspoons calcium water (packet comes with pectin)

juice of 1/4 lemon

Grind or purée peppers in blender or food processor with 3 tablespoons water. Add stevia to taste. Pour into a bowl. Prepare calcium water and stir into pepper mixture. Bring 1/2 cup water just to a boil and pour into food processor or blender. Quickly add pectin and lemon juice and blend. (You must work fast, or the pectin will form globs.) Quickly pour pectin mixture into bowl with pepper mixture and stir well. Pour into glass jar and refrigerate. It will gel completely in a couple hours.

Red Pepper Jelly

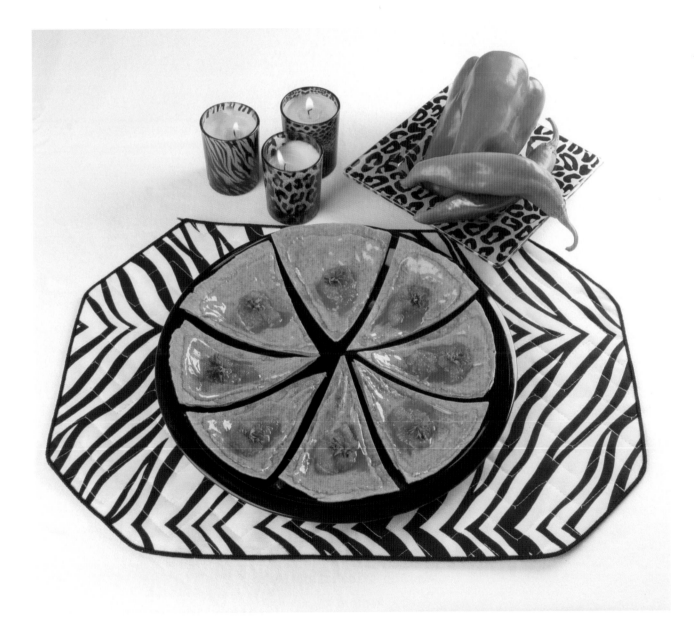

Avocado Coconut Key Lime Pie

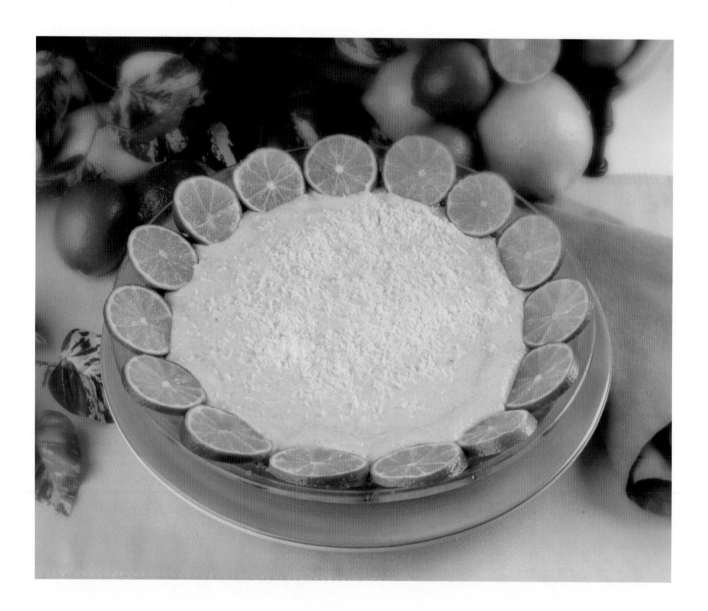

"Avocado is God's butter."
Shelley Redford Young

Avocado Coconut Key Lime Pie

By Debra Jenkins. 1st place Transitional recipes, The pH Miracle Recipe Contest.

Add all ingredients (except the psyllium flakes and lime peel) to a food processor or blender and mix till smooth and creamy. Add more stevia to taste. Fold in psyllium flakes and lime peel. Spoon into already prepared Almond Nut Pie Crust. Sprinkle coconut and chopped walnuts or pecans over top as garnish and chill in refrigerator for 1–2 hours.

Variation by Shelley: Add 6 tablespoons coconut milk to the first batch of ingredients, and reduce psyllium to 1 tablespoon.

8 oz. Silken Tofu

1/2 cup fresh lime juice

1 teaspoon Frontier non-alcoholic vanilla

2 tablespoons fresh grated coconut

1/8 teaspoon Real Salt

1 small or 1/2 medium avocado

1/8 teaspoon powdered white stevia

1/8 teaspoon lime peel, grated

3 tablespoons psyllium flakes (or agar flakes)

Almond Nut Pie Crust

By Debra Jenkins. 1st place, Transitional recipes, for The pH Miracle Recipe Contest.

Combine dry ingredients in a mixing bowl. Combine the water, melted butter and vanilla and pour over dry ingredients. Mix well. Transfer mixture to a 9" pie plate. Press mixture firmly into place with your fingers, making sure to cover bottom and sides of pie plate. For an unfilled pie crust, bake empty pie shell at 350 degrees for 18–20 minutes or until lightly brown. Cool and fill with pie filling. For a filled pie crust, first bake the empty crust for 10 minutes, then fill and finish baking pie per recipe.

Variation: Replace flax meal with ground coconut.

1/2 cup fresh spelt flakes ground into flour (I use my old coffee grinder)

1/2 cup ground almonds

1/4 cup fresh ground flax meal

1 tablespoon arrowroot powder

1/2 teaspoon ground cinnamon

1/8 teaspoon ground cloves

1 packet stevia powder

1 teaspoon Frontier alcohol-free vanilla

2 tablespoons Garden of Life coconut butter (melted)

2 tablespoons water

Deliciously Dill Petaled Cucumbers

2 English cucumbers

1 teaspoon Deliciously Dill Seasoning (Spice Hunter)

juice of 1 large lime

small amount of water, if needed

Real Salt, to taste

Run fork prongs along each cucumber to create a petaled look, then slice them 1/4 inch thick. Place sliced cucumber in shallow bowl with juice, dill seasoning and salt. Marinate in the fridge for at least half an hour. Serve chilled.

Pumpkin Cream Pie

By Debra Jenkins. 1st place transitional recipes, in The pH Miracle Recipe Contest. Serves 6–8.

1 pkg. Silken Tofu (12 oz.)

2 cups fresh pureed pumpkin (or yams)

2 teaspoons Frontier alcohol-free vanilla

2 teaspoons cinnamon

1/4 teaspoon Real Salt

3/4 teaspoon nutmeg

1/4 teaspoon cloves

1/2 teaspoon ginger

1/4 teaspoon white stevia powder (or 2–3 packets stevia with fiber powder)

3 tablespoons psyllium (agar powder or flakes can be substituted for psyllium)

Mix tofu, pumpkin, vanilla, cinnamon, salt, nutmeg, cloves, ginger and stevia powder together in a food processor till smooth and creamy. (Add more spices or stevia if you like, or use less spices for a milder pie). Lastly, add psyllium and blend. Scoop into prepared Almond Nut Pie Crust (page 109) and chill for at least an hour. Top with Nutty Crème Topping or Tofu Whip Cream.

AB&J Sandwiches

By Cheri Freeman. 3rd place, the pH Miracle Recipe Contest. Serves 1–2.

sprouted wheat tortillas

almond Butter

Red Pepper Jelly (see p. 106)

Warm the tortillas and cut into quarters. Spread on Almond butter and red pepper jelly.

Makes little triangle sandwiches, a great snack!

Holiday Almonds

By JoAnn Efeney. Serves 2–4.

Put almonds into the water and add the spices. Let mixture set overnight, stir and enjoy.

Variation by Shelley: After almonds soak in the spices, drain and dehydrate. You'll get a nice extra-crunchy snack with a hint of spiciness.

1 cup water
1/2 cup almonds
1/8 teaspoon ground cloves
1/8 teaspoon ground ginger
1/8 teaspoon ground nutmeg
1/8 teaspoon ground cinnamon

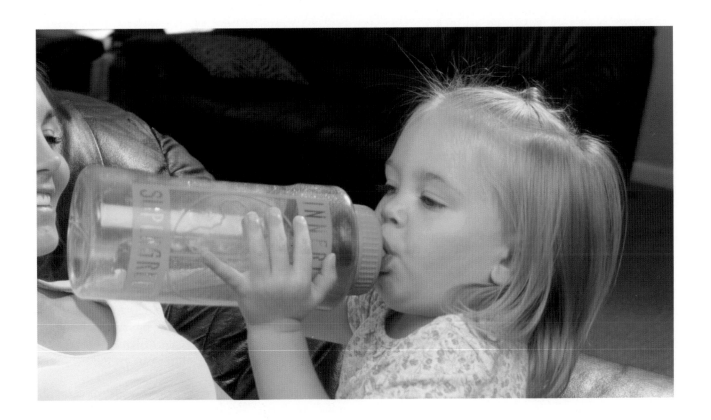

Veggie Crispy Crackers with Soy Sprouts Powder

These are great for a crunchy cracker snack, or broken up and sprinkled over a salad like croutons.

3 carrots

1 small carton of cherry or grape tomatoes

3 sun dried tomatoes packed in olive oil

1 teaspoon fresh ginger

3 stalks celery

2 tomatillos

1/3 yam, peeled

1 yellow neck squash

1/3 cup fresh mixed herbs, such as rosemary, oregano, tarragon, thyme, cilantro, parsley, and basil

1/2 cup sprouted buckwheat (I use a two day sprout—soak raw buckwheat for 6–8 hours and rinse for two days)

1/3 cup flax seeds (you don't have to soak them)

1–2 heaping tablespoons soy sprouts powder

Put first nine ingredients into your food processor and pulse chop until all veggies are mixed well, moist, and diced. Or, if you prefer, place all nine ingredients through the Green Power juicer with the blank attachment and put moist pulp into a mixing bowl. Add the sprouted buckwheat, flax seeds, and soy powder and mix well. Pour mixture out onto plastic sheet-lined trays for the dehydrator and pat or spatula the mixture out into a large square or rectangle. Dehydrate for 4–5 hours at 90–95 degrees, and then cut into smaller squares (3x3 inches) and transfer to the mesh-lined trays for continued drying until crisp (about 4 hours more). Or, let the crackers continue drying through the night and break the finished pieces up into small pieces in the morning. If done right, these can last up to a month in an air tight container, though I'm sure they will be eaten up long before that!

Bird Nest Crackers

These are fun to place on the top of a bowl of soup right before you serve it. I form these crackers into little nest shapes and put some fresh peas from the pod in them for hors d'oeuvres. Plain, these crackers travel well. Being dehydrated, they offer concentrated nutrition.

2 yellow crook neck squash, shredded

2 zucchini, shredded

1/2 teaspoon Real Salt

1/2 teaspoon Chef's All Purpose Shake (Spice Hunter) or seasoning of choice

2 teaspoons Vegetable Seasoning (Spice Hunter) or seasoning of choice

Clean squash and zucchini, taking care to cut any scars off of the skin. Shred in food processor and combine with spices. Spoon out onto Teflon sheets. You can make the crackers more lacey by loosely placing the mixture on the sheet in a small circle which will dry like a lacey cracker with holes showing, or you can pack the mixture tightly and form little nests to create a denser cracker nest. Dehydrate overnight to 24 hours and store in an air tight container.

Variation: Experiment with added veggies, seeds or nuts like soaked almonds, sunflower seeds, sweet peas, shredded carrots, jalapenos, and flax seeds. You can also use your own favorite seasonings to get the flavors you like best.

"God has the most incredible wrappers! The pea's pod . . . the tomatillo's paper skin sheath . . . the artichoke's shields that protect it's heart . . . God is too cool!"

Shelley Redford Young

Veggie Crispy Crackers with Soy Sprouts Powder

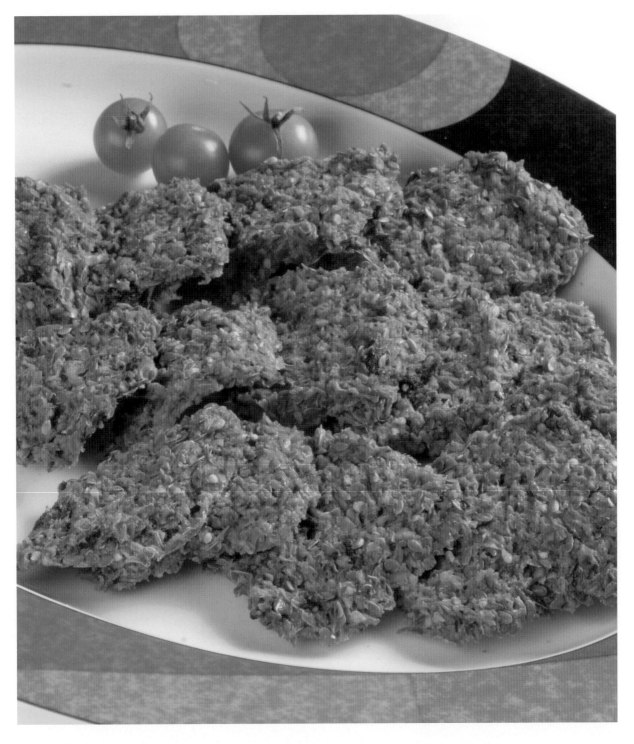

Veggie Crispy Crackers with Soy Sprouts Powder

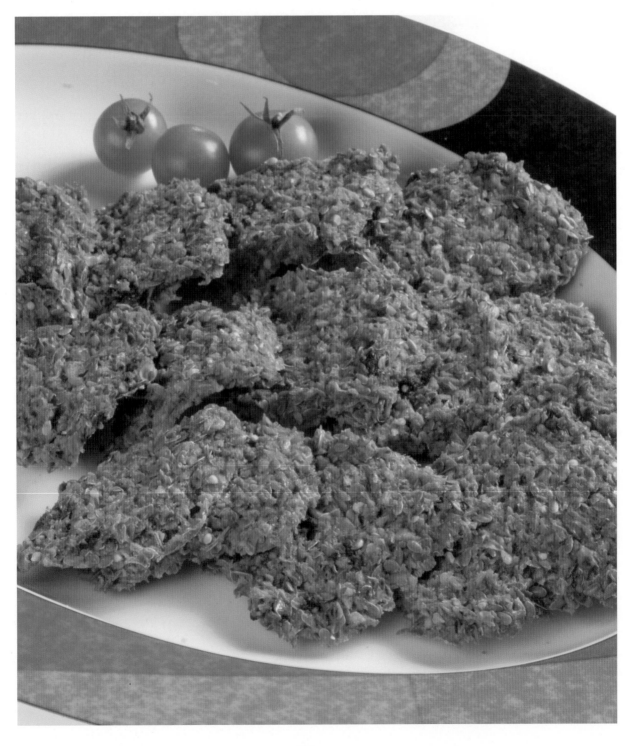

Super Soy Pudding

This is a great way to have a delicious snack while staying alkaline. We even eat this wonderful pudding for breakfast or in place of one of the soups on the cleanse. It is high is good fats, vitamin E, Calcium, and Potassium with the almond milk and avocado, and high in good proteins from the Super Soy Powder. Serves 2.

1 cup Fresh Silky Almond Milk (see recipe on p. 36) or coconut milk.
1 avocado
1 whole lime, peeled
2 scoops sprouted soy powder
1 pkg. stevia
6–8 ice cubes

Put all ingredients in a blender and blend on high until rich and smooth and pudding like.

Variations:
* Coconut Super Soy Pudding: Use the coconut milk, and add 2 tablespoons unsweetened dried coconut granules to the mix. Sprinkle some coconut over the top before serving.

* Lemon Super Soy Pudding: Use a lemon instead of a lime.

* Grapefruit Super Soy Pudding: Use juice from 1/2 grapefruit instead of lime.

* Super Green Super Soy Pudding: Add 1/2 scoop of green powder or 1 cup fresh baby spinach.

* Ginger Super Soy Pudding: Add a pinch or two of fresh grated ginger

* Cinnamon Super Soy Pudding: Add a pinch or two of cinnamon and nutmeg to the mix, and sprinkle more on top.

* Nutty Super Soy Pudding: Add chopped raw almonds (or pecans or macadamias, or whatever you like)

* Super Soy Pops: Pour your favorite variation into pop molds and freeze. Or use small paper cups or ice cube trays, with pop sticks or toothpicks added when partially frozen.

* Super Soy Slushy: Freeze your favorite variation in ice cube trays, thaw slightly, and chop up.

Edamame Beans

Edamame is the Japanese word for soybeans. Put the whole pod into your mouth, bite down and slide out the beans for a yummy snack or side dish.

Boil the edamame as per the directions on the package. Strain, then dash with a few squirts of olive oil and some Real Salt or favorite Spice Hunter seasonings. We like Vegetable Rub or Garlic Herb Bread Seasoning (Spice Hunter). Good served warm or cold.

1 package frozen edamame (soy beans)
oil
Real Salt
Seasoning of your choice

Super Soy Pudding

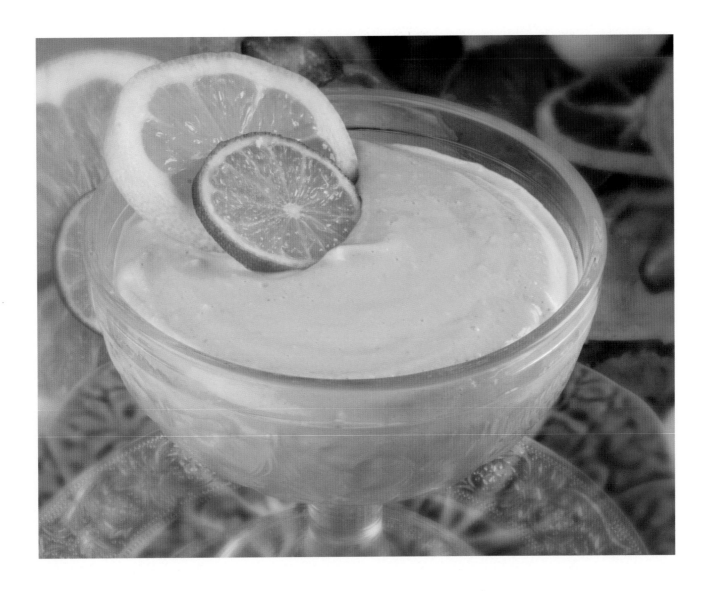

Sprouted Buckwheat Flatties

These are thin and crust-like in texture. They are marvelous as a raw (low heat dehydrated) pizza crust. You can dry them big in large rounds or break them up and use them as crackers or sandwich pieces. Experiment with this basic recipe and come up with versions of your own! You will need a good dehydrator, a food processor and sprouting equipment. The preparation for these flatties may seem like a lot of time and work, but once you get the hang of it, it will surely be worth it! I triple and quadruple this recipe to fill my entire Excalibur (nine trays) with flatties. They will stay fresh in a zip-lock bag or Tupperware for as long as a month. Great for hiking and camping trips, biking, or on a long flight. Our grandson CharLee is cutting his first teeth on these alkaline crackers!

3 cups sprouted buckwheat (I use a two day sprout—soak raw buckwheat for 6–8 hours and rinse for two days)

1/3 cup Essential Balance Oil (Omega Nutrition or Arrowhead Mills)

2 teaspoons Garlic Herb Bread Seasonings (Spice Hunter)

2 teaspoons Real Salt

1 teaspoon All Purpose Chef's Shake (Spice Hunter)

1 1/3 cup carrot pulp or shredded carrot, or raw yam, squash or zucchini, or a mixture of those

2–3 sun dried tomatoes (optional)

1/3–2/3 cup flax seeds (you don't have to soak)

1/4–1/3 cup water (optional)

Pulse chop veggie pulp, oil, salt, and seasonings in a food processor to mix well. Then add remaining ingredients and continue to process until you get a thick batter that is quite smooth. (You could also stop mixing earlier if you would prefer a coarse batter with more whole buckwheat sprouts.) While the food processor is running, you can add the water if you feel the batter needs to be thinned some to make spreading easier. Pour or scoop mixture out onto plastic-lined trays for dehydration. Use a spatula to help spread out the batter so your flattie is 1/4 to 1/2 inch thick. Dehydrate at 90–100 degrees overnight or 7–8 hours. Carefully lift the flatties and transfer them to a mesh-lined tray and continue dehydrating until totally crisp and dry, about 4–6 more hours.

Variation: Experiment with other seasonings in place of the Chef's Shake. For example: 1 tablespoon soy sprouts powder, 1 teaspoon green powder, Italian pizza seasoning, 2 tablespoons fresh basil, or whatever you like best.

Appendix A: Resources

Foods You Should Never Eat

Here are Dr. Robert O. Young's top 16 foods that you should never eat, drink or inhale if you want to prevent disease and imbalance symptomologies like diabetes.

- All dairy including milk, cottage cheese, cheese, butter and yogurt
- All meats including pork, beef, chicken, turkey and lamb
- All fermented foods or condiments including soy sauce, vinegar, sauerkraut, miso, olives, horseradish, tamari, mayonnaise, salad dressings, mustard, ketchup, steak sauce, monosodium glutamate (MSG)and tempeh
- All grains including rice, wheat, barley, oats, cereals, pasta, pastries, etc.
- All fruit except for the exceptions already mentioned
- All legumes unless sprouted
- All acidic drinks like coffee, tea and soda pop
- All alcohol including beer and wine no exceptions
- Root vegetables like potato and yams
- All sugars and sweets, especially chocolate
- Corn or corn products
- Salted or processed nuts, especially peanuts
- Edible fungus or mushrooms (this also includes baker's or brewers yeast and algae)
- NO processed foods, period! These foods are also called non-foods or junk foods
- Smoking and/or chewing tobacco
- Heated or processed oil

Microorganism/pathological load comparisons in foods:

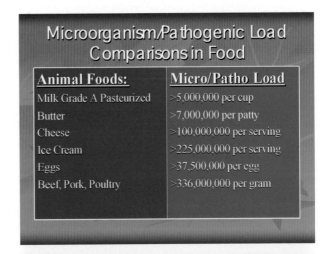

Animal Foods:	Micro/Patho Load
Milk Grade A Pasteurized	>5,000,000 per cup
Butter	>7,000,000 per patty
Cheese	>100,000,000 per serving
Ice Cream	>225,000,000 per serving
Eggs	>37,500,000 per egg
Beef, Pork, Poultry	>336,000,000 per gram

Microorganism/Pathogenic Load Comparisons in Food

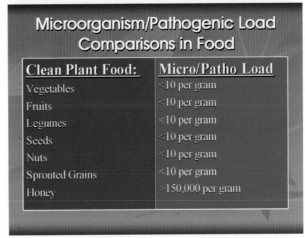

Clean Plant Food:	Micro/Patho Load
Vegetables	<10 per gram
Fruits	<10 per gram
Legumes	<10 per gram
Seeds	<10 per gram
Nuts	<10 per gram
Sprouted Grains	<10 per gram
Honey	>150,000 per gram

Microorganism/Pathogenic Load Comparisons in Food

The average American meal of animal proteins, eggs and dairy contains over 750,000,000 to 1,000,000,000 biological transmutations per meal (US Department of Agriculture).

The average vegetarian meal consisting of only plant foods has less than 500 biological transmutations per meal.

Dr. Robert O. Young's Top 11 Foods to Eat Freely

For a healthy and energetic body free of sickness and disease and especially free of diabetes:

- All varieties of avocado (there are over 400) and avocado oil
- Unsweetened coconut and coconut oil
- Lemon, lime, and grapefruit
- All varieties of tomato
- Wheat grass and barley grass
- All the green vegetables that grow above the ground, including broccoli, spinach, celery, kale, cucumber, parsley, and leafy greens, especially dandelion

- Sprouts like bean, mung, broccoli, soy, radish and sunflower
- Nuts and nut milks like almond and hazelnuts
- Seeds like flax, borage, sunflower, buckwheat and sesame
- Cold pressed oils of olive, fax, primrose, borage, and hemp
- Fresh water and cold water fish like trout, salmon, tuna, mackerel, and eel

Product/Organization Information

Spice Hunter Spices
San Luis Obispo, CA 93401
800-444-3061
www.spicehunter.com

Vita Mix Blenders
8615 Usher Road
Cleveland, Ohio 44138-2199
800 848-2649
www.vita-mix.com

Green Power Juicers
Orders: 888-254-7336
Inquiries: 562-940-4241
Fax: 562-940-4240
www.greenpower.com

Organic Food-Mail Order
Diamond Organics
P.O. Box 2159
Freedom, CA 95019
Shop toll-free: 888-674-2642
Shop by Fax: 888-888-6777
Organics@diamondorganics.com

Life Sprouts
P.O. Box 150
Paradise, Utah 94321
435-245-3891
www.lifesprouts.net

Cutco Knives
www.cutco.com

Real Salt@
Redmond Minerals, Inc.
800-367-7258
www.realsalt.com

Coconut Oil (Extra Virgin)
Wilderness Family Naturals
Box 538 Finland MN 55603
1-866-936-6457 or
1-218-220-0762
www.wildernessfamilynaturals.com

Organic Coconut Oil
Omega Nutrition USA Inc.
1-800-661-FLAX

www.thepHmiracle.us
Dr. Young and Shelley's website with info on new recipes, New Biology microscopy courses, pH miracle retreats, and much more!

www.thepHmiraclecenter.com
Publications and other resources with the same info as thepHmiracle.us

www.InnerLightmotion.com
Dr. Robert and Shelley's newest website featuring video productions of product training, science, and lifestyle for the New Biology. Weekly episodes with the Young's featured. A wealth of information.

The pH Miracle Center
1-760-751-8321
email: info@thepHmiracle.us
fax: 1-760-751-8324
A clearing house of many products and information for products used in the *Back to the House of Health* books 1 and 2.

The InnerLight Foundation
A non-profit organization for donations, education, and information.
1-760-751-8321

Metric Conversion Chart

IMPERIAL	METRIC
1 inch	2.54 centimeters
1 ounce	28.35 grams
1 pound	0.45 kilogram
1/2 teaspoon	1.25 milliliters
1/2 teaspoon	2.5 milliliters
1 teaspoon	5 milliliters
1 tablespoon	15 milliliters
1/3 cup	80 milliliters
1/2 cup	120 milliliters
1 cup	250 milliliters
1 pint (2 cups)	480 milliliters
1 quart (4 cups; 32 ounces)	960 milliliters
1 gallon (4 quarts)	3.84 liters
16 fluid ounces	0.47 liter
32° Fahrenheit	0* Celsius

Note: Conversions in this book from imperial to metric are not exact. They have been rounded to the nearest standard measure for convenience. To prepare recipes more exactly, follow the imperial measures.

Glossary of Terms

Acid: A compound capable of donating a hydrogen ion (proton) to a base. A product of fermentation by microforms, degenerative to body substances, cells and tissues.

Aduki bean: A legume, also called "adzuki bean." The small seeds of a bushy annual plant native to China, aduki beans are a popular ingredient in Chinese and Japanese cooking.

Agar: Gelling and thickening agent of plant origin, made from the cell wall of red algae.

Alkaline: Relating to, containing, or having the reaction of an alkali base.

Almonds: Particularly rich in protein, iron, calcium, vitamin B2 and vitamin E. Almonds make a very good milk, and butter when ground. Soaking hydrates them for a wonderful crunchy snack.

Ash residue: The by-product of food and energy metabolism, which can be neutral, acid, or alkaline.

Amino acids: The constituents of proteins, eight of which are essential to the human body. Without them, severe metabolic and growth disorders result.

Black beans: Kidney shaped with a shiny skin and white center, these beans are grown widely in South America. Sometimes called "turtle beans."

Brazil nuts: Rich in protein, the B vitamin thiamine, and magnesium. Brazil nuts have a creamy texture and a delicate flavor that makes them excellent for eating raw in salads or snacks.

Buckwheat: Not a cereal but rather a simple variety of bistort with triangular seeds whose contents are nonetheless like those of a cereal. Contains protein and many minerals as well as lysine, an essential amino acid that rarely occurs in cereals. Buckwheat is desirable because it contains no gluten and is considered low fungal.

Celery Root: (known as Celeriac) is different from celery although the taste is a bit similiar. Celery root is a large gnarly rough skinned root.(not the most attractive of vegetables in the produce section) and, a very good potassium and natural sodium-rich food that is good for thickening soups and gravys.

Chlorophyll: The green coloring in plants, chlorophyll plays an essential role in photosynthesis and is thought to be a genuine elixir of health.

Coconut meat: the pudding like substance found in Young or Thai coconuts. High in Fosphorus for aid in building bones, and other essential fatty oils to contribute to sound health

Coconut Milk: the meat and the water of a Young or Thai coconut blended together.

Coconut water: clear water like fluid from the Young or Thai coconut. It has the same or near same pH as the blood at 7.36..and is high in Lauric Oils that are so beneficial to sound health. A natural anti-fungal and anti- microbial liquid. Used in many of the Back to the House of Health 2 recipes as a fluid to boost shakes, puddings, popcycles, or to steam fish or veggies in.

Cranberry beans: Also known as "Shelly beans" in Indiana and Ohio. This bean has a much sweeter and more delicate flavor than the pinto bean. When cooked it loses its markings and becomes solid in color. Great in soups, side dishes, and pasta dishes.

Flax seeds: Flax seeds are very high in omega-3 and omega-6 essential fats. They are available in most health-food stores. They can be ground or soaked, and are used also as a thickener.

Food combining: Nutritional fundamental rules for combining compatible foods together for optimum health.

Garbanzo beans: An annual bush with short pods; its beans are light beige-yellow. Used in Africa, Spain and India to make flour, hummus, purees, stews and vegetable accompaniments. Also known as chickpeas.

Hazelnuts: A good source of vitamin E and low in fat, also known as "filberts." Hazelnuts can also be soaked like almonds.

Kamut: An older cereal variety from Ancient Egypt with grains often three times the size of wheat. High protein content as well as being rich in amino acids and vitamins. Provides a robust nutty flavor.

Kidney beans: Red color and kidney shape make these beans distinctive, as does their fine aroma. Very popular in South America. Very high in fiber and good for soups and salads.

Kuzu Root: Also known as "kudzu." A natural jelling and thickening agent made from a root that grows wild in Japan.

Lentils: Small legumes, rich in protein, iron, calcium, and B vitamins. Can be used for sprouting. Available in many colors, green and red being the most common.

Macadamia nuts: These nuts are expensive and very creamy. They are usually sold roasted and salted. Try to buy them raw and freeze them for a longer shelf life.

Microzyma: An organized ferment. An independently living, imperishable fundamental anatomical element. Capable of multiplying, it is the basic form from which organisms are constituted, and to which they are reduced upon death.

Microforms: A general term for microscopic life forms. It covers everything from microzymas to mold, beneficial to harmful.

Millet: The oldest cultivated variety of cereal in the world and an important basic foodstuff in Africa and Central Asia, as well as being used widely in Europe. Very rich in unsaturated fatty acids and vitamins and good as a rice substitute.

Monounsaturated fats: Generally found in oil, they are present in practically all foods that contain fat, both animal and vegetable. They are generally liquid at room temperature and can be metabolized by the body. They are used mainly as good energy-burning fat in the body.

Mung beans: Cultivated in China and India, where they are known as "mungdal." They are also made into bean sprouts.

Nori: Popular green seaweed that comes in square sheet, used for making sushi.

Olive oil: This oil is mostly associated with Mediterranean cuisine, and is easily digested and has a positive effect on the stomach and intestines. It is also known to reduce the risk of heart and circulatory diseases. It has a broad range of flavors, depending on the type of olive, time of harvest, the climate, and type of soil. It should not be refrigerated but should be stored in a cool, dark place. It keeps very well for nine to twelve months.

Pecans: Pecans offer a delicious mealy texture which is good in salads, wraps, and warmed nut loafs. They can also be soaked with good results.

pH: The symbol expressing the degree of alkalinity or acidity of a solution. A solution with pH of 7 is neutral; values below 7 indicate a degree of acidity; values above 7 indicate a degree of alkalinity. The normal pH of blood serum is approximately 7.3 and the normal pH of the urine is 6.8.

Pinenuts: Protein-rich pinenuts, also known as "pignoli" or "piñons," are soft, white, creamy-colored nuts taken from the pine cone of the piñon tree. Store in the freezer, as these nuts have a very short shelf-life.

Pleomorphism: The principle that microforms are not fixed species, as are higher animals and plants, but can rapidly change both form and function during a life cycle. The occurrence of various shapes in the same developmental phase or form.

Polyunsaturated fats: Like linoleic acid (bi-saturated), linolenic acid (tri-saturated) and arachidon acid (vitamin F). Usually vegetable fats, they are liquid, react easily and are essential for human organisms. They help the body regulate all its functions, and as the body cannot produce these fats, they are an important part of the diet.

Pumpkin seeds: Sometimes called "pita seeds," pumpkin seeds are particularly rich in minerals, especially zinc. They are a good addition to any meal. Soaking plumps them and softens their taste.

Quinoa: A plant that grows in the Andes at altitudes in excess of 13,000 feet (4000 meters). Nutritious as a leaf vegetable and having small seeds rich in vitamins and other nutrients, it was much prized by the Incas. When used as flour, it can be bitter because it contains saporin. Mostly available in health food stores.

Rice: Asia's main foodstuff that loses its nutrients when milled and polished to produce white rice. However, Basmati rice is a naturally occurring white rice. Hulled, natural brown rice or whole-grain rice contain all eight essential amino acids, vitamins and minerals. Because of extensive use of pesticides, it is advisable only to use organic, whole-grain rice.

Saturated fats: These include palmitin, stearin and butyric acid. They are found in all animal fats and also in palm and coconut oil; additionally, they are produced in the human body. They are often solid at room temperature, do not react and are very hard to digest.

Sesame seeds: Rich in B3, iron, protein and zinc, sesame seeds are usually white but may be brown, red or black, depending on the variety. Tahini is a butter made from ground sesame seeds.

Spelt: This form of wheat has highly nutritious gluten and is recommended as a good alternative grain, since virtually all spelt is grown organically.

Stevia: (Stevia Rebaudiana) also known as "sweet herb". A plant indigenous to mountainous regions of Brazil and Paraguay. A small perennial shrub with green leaves that belongs to the aster or chrysanthemum family of plants. It's common form is know as stevioside, a fine white powder extracted from the leaves of the plant. It has a sweetening rate between 70-400 times that of white sugar, completely calorie free, never inititating a rise in blood sugar and does not provide food for micro organisms like bacteria and yeasts. It contains no artificial ingredients.

Sunflower seeds: Nutritionally speaking, sunflower seeds are a good source of vitamins B1, B6, and potassium. They also produce a hearty sprout that is high in protein.

Super Soy Sprouts: Dehydrated, organically grown baby soy sprouts

Tofu: Soybean product obtained by coagulation.

Tomatillo: a tart tomato like fruit grown in Mexico for seasoning food. Has a green-apple tomato flavor. Great in salsas, shakes or snacks. Comes with a papery husk that you simply peel off before using.

UDO's: The brand name for an oil blend developed by Udo Erasmus, author of *Fats that Heal, Fats that Kill*. A blend of unrefined oils consisting of flax, sunflower, sesame and evening primrose. Found in the refrigerated sections of most health food stores.